Practical Manual of

PHARMACEUTICS-II

For

Second Year Diploma Pharmacy Students
(According to PCI, ER 1991)

DR. G. D. GUPTA (M. Pharm. Ph. D, MBA)
DIRECTOR-CUM-PRINCIPAL
ISF COLLEGE OF PHARMACY, MOGA, PUNJAB.

DR. SHAILESH SHARMA (M. Pharm. Ph. D,)
PRINCIPAL
ASBASJSM DIPLOMA COLLEGE OF PHARMACY, BELA (ROPAR) PUNJAB.

NEELAM SHARMA (M. Pharm.)
ASSISTANT PROFESSOR (PHARMACEUTICS)
ASBASJSM COLLEGE OF PHARMACY, BELA (ROPAR) PUNJAB.

Name:____

Roll No.:____

Session:____

College Name:____

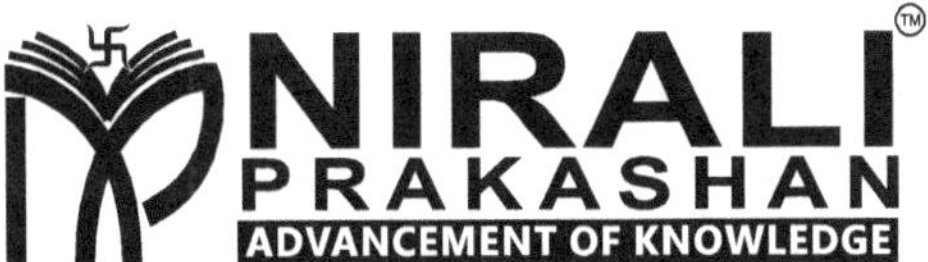

N2587

PHARMACEUTICS-II   **ISBN 978-93-86700-55-1**

Fourth Edition   :   **February 2020**

©   :   **Authors**

Published By :

NIRALI PRAKASHAN

Abhyudaya Pragati, 1312, Shivaji Nagar

Off J.M. Road, PUNE – 411005

Tel - (020) 25512336/37/39, Fax - (020) 25511379

Email : niralipune@pragationline.com

➤ DISTRIBUTION CENTRES

PUNE

Nirali Prakashan : 119, Budhwar Peth, Jogeshwari Mandir Lane, Pune 411002, Maharashtra
(For orders within Pune)   Tel : (020) 2445 2044, 66022708, Mobile : 9657703145
   Email : niralilocal@pragationline.com

Nirali Prakashan : S. No. 28/27, Dhayari, Near Asian College Pune 411041
(For orders outside Pune)   Tel : (020) 24690204 Fax : (020) 24690316; Mobile : 9657703143
   Email : bookorder@pragationline.com

MUMBAI

Nirali Prakashan : 385, S.V.P. Road, Rasdhara Co-op. Hsg. Society Ltd.,
   Girgaum, Mumbai 400004, Maharashtra; Mobile : 9320129587
   Tel : (022) 2385 6339 / 2386 9976, Fax : (022) 2386 9976
   Email : niralimumbai@pragationline.com

➤ DISTRIBUTION BRANCHES

JALGAON

Nirali Prakashan : 34, V. V. Golani Market, Navi Peth, Jalgaon 425001, Maharashtra,
   Tel : (0257) 222 0395, Mob : 94234 91860; Email : niralijalgaon@pragationline.com

KOLHAPUR

Nirali Prakashan : New Mahadvar Road, Kedar Plaza, 1st Floor Opp. IDBI Bank, Kolhapur 416 012
   Maharashtra. Mob : 9850046155; Email : niralikolhapur@pragationline.com

NAGPUR

Nirali Prakashan : Above Maratha Mandir, Shop No. 3, First Floor,
   Rani Jhanshi Square, Sitabuldi, Nagpur 440012, Maharashtra
   Tel : (0712) 254 7129; Email : niralinagpur@pragationline.com

DELHI

Nirali Prakashan : 4593/15, Basement, Agarwal Lane, Ansari Road, Daryaganj
   Near Times of India Building, New Delhi 110002 Mob : 08505972553
   Email : niralidelhi@pragationline.com

BENGALURU

Nirali Prakashan : Maitri Ground Floor, Jaya Apartments, No. 99, 6th Cross, 6th Main,
   Malleswaram, Bengaluru 560003, Karnataka; Mob : 9449043034
   Email: niralibangalore@pragationline.com

Other Branches : Hyderabad, Chennai

niralipune@pragationline.com | www.pragationline.com

Also find us on [f] www.facebook.com/niralibooks

CERTIFICATE

This is to certify that Mr. /Ms. _________________________________

is a regular student of _____________________________________

D. Pharmacy Second Year. He/She has completed his/her

practical work of Pharmaceutics-II in the supervision of

Dr./Mr./Ms. ______________________ during the academic session

201___/201___.

Number of practicals performed _________ out of _________ in the

subject of Pharmaceutics-II.

Roll No. ________________

Date:____/_____/________

Signature of Student

Teacher In-charge

Principal Signature

Institute Rubber Stamp

Syllabus ...

THEORY **(75 Hours)**

1. Dispensing Pharmacy:
   - (i) Prescriptions-Reading and understanding of prescription; Latin terms commonly used (Detailed study is not necessary), Modern methods of prescribing, adoption of metric system. Calculations involved in dispensing.
   - (ii) Incompatibilities in Prescriptions-Study of various types of incompatibilities-physical, chemical and therapeutic.
   - (iii) Posology-Dose and Dosage of drugs, Factors influencing dose, Calculations of doses on the basis of age, sex and surface area. Veterinary doses.

2. Dispensed Medications:
   (Note: A detailed study of the following dispensed medication is necessary. Methods of preparation with theoretical and practical aspects, use of appropriate containers and closures. Special labelling requirements and storage conditions should be high-lighted).
   - (i) Powders-Types of powders-Advantages and disadvantages of powders, Granules, Cachets and Tablet triturates. Preparation of different types of powders encountered in prescriptions. Weighing methods, possible errors in weighing, minimum weighable amounts and weighing of material below the minimum weighable amount, geometric dilution and proper usage and care of dispensing balance.
   - (ii) Liquid Oral Dosage Forms:
   - (a) Monophasic-Theoretical aspects including commonly used vehicles, essential adjuvants like stabilizers, colourants and flavours, with examples.
     Review of the following monophasic liquids with details of formulation and practical methods.

Liquids for internal administration	Liquids for external administration or used on mucus membranes.
Mixtures and concentrates	Gargles
Syrups	Mouth washes Throat-paints Douches
Elixirs	Ear Drops Nasal drops & Sprays Liniments Lotions.

   - (b) Biphasic Liquid Dosage Forms:
   - (i) Suspension (elementary study)----Suspensions containing diffusible solids and liquids and their preparations. Study of the adjuvants used like thickening agents, wetting agents, their necessity and quantity to be incorporated. Suspensions of precipitate forming liquids like, tinctures, their preparations and stability. Suspensions produced by chemical reaction. An introduction to flocculated, non-flocculated suspension system.
   - (ii) Emulsions-Types of emulsions, identification of emulsion system, formulation of emulsions, selection of emulsifying agents. Instabilities in emulsions. Preservation of emulsions.
   - (iii) Semi-Solid Dosage Forms:
   - (a) Ointments-Types of ointments, classification and selection of dermatological vehicles. Preparation and stability of ointments by the following processes:
   - (i) Trituration (ii) Fusion (iii) Chemical reaction (iv) Emulsification.
   - (b) Pastes--- Difference between ointments and pastes, bases of pastes. Preparation of pastes and their preservation.
   - (c) Jellies-An introduction to the different types of jellies and their preparation.
   - (d) An elementary study of poultice.
   - (e) Suppositories and pessaries-Their relative merits and demerits, types of suppositories, suppository bases, classification, properties, Preparation and packing of suppositories. Use of suppositories for drug absorption.
   - (iv) Dental and Cosmetic Preparations: Introduction to Dentrifices, Facial cosmetics, Deodorants, Antiperspirants, Shampoos, Hair dressing and Hair removers.
   - (v) Sterile Dosage Forms:
   - (a) Parenteral dosage forms-Definitions, General requirements for parenteral dosage forms. Types of parenteral formulations, vehicles, adjuvants, processing, personnel, facilities and Quality control. Preparation of Intravenous fluids and admixtures-Total parenteral nutrition, Dialysis fluids.
   - (b) Sterility testing, Particulate matter monitoring-Faulty seal packaging.
   - (c) Ophthalmic Products-Study of essential characteristics of different ophthalmic preparations. Formulation additives, special precautions in handling and storage of ophthalmic products.

PRACTICAL **(100 Hours)**

Dispensing of at least 100 products covering a wide range of preparations such as mixtures, emulsions, lotions, liniments, E.N.T, preparations, ointments, suppositories, powders, incompatible prescriptions etc.

❖ ❖ ❖

CLASSIFICATION OF DOSAGE FORM

According to Type of Dosage Form :

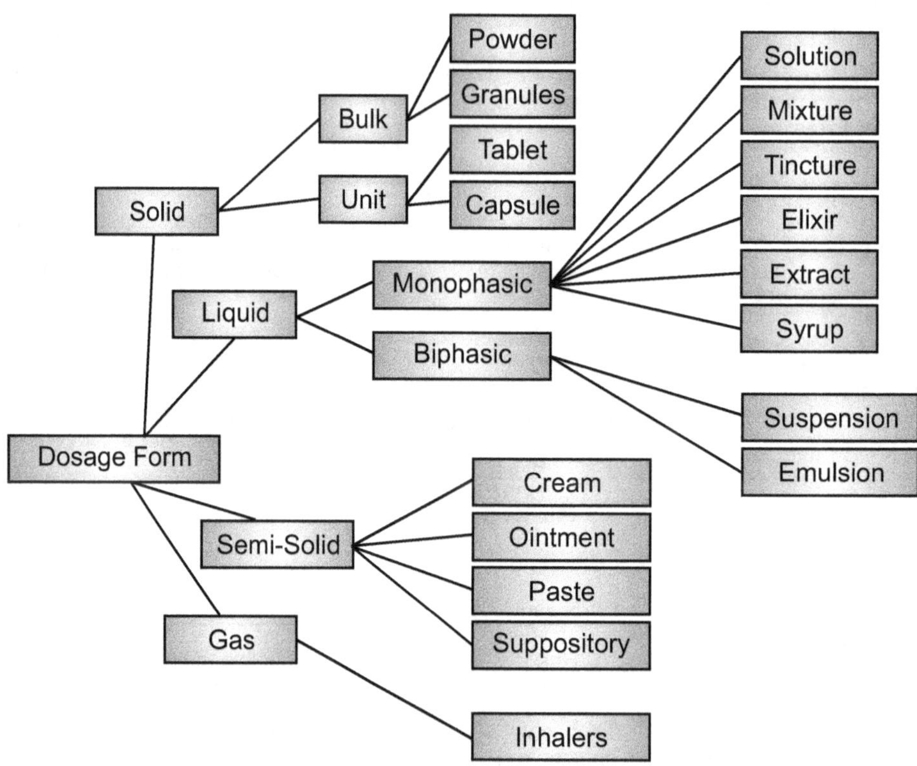

According to Route of Drug Administration :

ROUTE			
	Oral	Solid	Tablet, Capsule, Powder
		Liquid	Syrup, Suspension, Emulsion
		Semi-solid	Jellies
	Topical	Solid	Powder
		Liquid	Lotion, Liniment
		Semi-solid	Cream, Ointment
	Parentral	Liquid	Injection, Infusion
	Inserts	Eye	Drop, Cream
		Nose	Drops
		Uretheral	Suppository

LATIN TERMS

Terms Related to Dosage Form

Abbreviation	Latin Term	Translation	Abbreviation	Latin Term	Translation
aurin.	Aurinarium	An ear cone	auristill.	Auristillae	Ear drop
buginar.	Buginarium	Nasal drop	caps. amylac.	Capsula amylacea	A cachet
caps.	Capsula	A capsule	caps. gelat.	Capsula gelatina	A gelatin capsule
cataplasm.	Cataplasma	A poultice	cereol.	Cereolus	An urethral bougie
collun.	Collunarium	A nosewash	collut.	Collutorium	A mouthwash
collyr.	Collyrium	An eye lotion	crem.	Cremor	A cream
emul.	Emulsion	An emulsion	garg.	Gargarisma	A gargle
gelat.	Gelatina	A jelly	gtt.	guttae	A drop
ht.	Haustus	A draught	inhal.	Inhalatio	An inhalation
insuff.	Insufflations	An insufflations	lin.	Linctus	A lictus
lin.	Linimemtum	A liniment	lot.	Lotio	A lotion
m., mist.	Mistura	A mixture	neb.	Nebula	A spray solution
oblat.	Oblatum	A cachet	past.	Pasta	A paste
pastill.	Pastillus	A pastille	pess.	Pessus	A pessary
pigm.	Pigmentum	A paint	pil.	Pills	A pill
pulv.	Pulvis	A powder	consper.	Consperus	A dusting powder
sternut	Sternutamentum	A snuff	suppose.	Suppositorium	A suppository
tab.	Tabletta	A tablet	troch.	Trochiscus	A lozenge
ung.	Unguentum	An ointment	n.p.	Nomen Proprium	Proper name

Terms used in preparation of dosage form

Abbreviation	Latin Term	Translation	Abbreviation	Latin Term	Translation
ft.	Fiat	Let be made	m.	Misce	Mix
m.ft.m.	Misce fiat mistura	Mix to make a mixture	div.	Divide	Divided
ter.	Tere	Rubbed	duplum.	Duplum	Twice the quantity
mitt.	Mitte	Send	dand.	Dandus	To be given
degult.	Deglutiendus	To be swallowed	infricand.	Infricandus	To be rubbed in
miscend.	Miscendus	To be mixed	sugend.	Sugendus	To be sucked
sum.	Sumendus	To be taken	u.a.	Ut antea	As before

Common terms used in Dose, Administration and Parts

Abbreviation	Latin Term	Translation	Abbreviation	Latin Term	Translation
b.i.d./b.d.	Bis in die	Twice a day	t.i.d./td	Ter in die	Three times a day
q.i.d./q.d.	Quarter in die	Four times a day	t.q.d.	Ter quaterve die	Three-four times a day
Prim.m.	Primo mane	Early in the morning	m.	Mane	In the morning
o.m.	Omni mane	Every morning	Jentac.	Jentaculum	Breakfast
o.n.	Omni nocte	Every night	h.d.	Hora decubitus	At bedtime
n.m.	Nocte maneque	Night and morning	o.h.	Omni hora	Every hour
o.alt.h	Omni altena hora	Every alternative hour	a.c.	Anti cibos	Before meals
a.c.	Anti cibum	Before food	p.c.	Post cibos	After food
i.c.	Inter cibos	Between meals	m.d.	More dicto	As directed
p.r.n.	Pro re nata	Occasionally	s.o.s.	Sis opus sit	When required
p.a.	Part affecta	To the affected part	sinsit.	Sinister	Left

MEASUREMENTS

Measure of Mass-Metric

1 tonne	1000 kilogram		1 quintol	1000 kilogram
1 kilogram	1000 gram		1 hectagram	100 gram
1 dekagram	10 gram		1 desigram	1/10 gram
1 centi gram	1/100 gram		1 milligram	1/1000 gram
1 microgram	10^{-6} gram		1 nanogram	10^{-9} gram
1 picogram	10^{-12} gram			

Measure of Length-Metric

1 kilometre	1000 meter		1 centimeter	1/100 meter
1 millimetre	1/1000 meter		1 micron	1/1000 meter
1 milli micron	10^{-6} mm		1 micro micron	10^{-9} mm

Measure of Capacity-Metric

1 hectolitre	100 litres		1 millilitre	1/1000 litre
1 litre	1000 millilitre		1 microlitre	10^{-6} litre
1000 litre	1 cubic litre			

Measures of mass- Imperial

1 ounce	437.5 grain		1 pound	16 ounces
1 stone	14 pound		1 hundred weight	112 pound
20 hundred weight	1 ton			

Measures of capacity (volume)- Imperial

60 minims	1 fluid drachum		8 fluid drachum	1 fluid ounce
20 fluid ounce	1 pint		2 pints	1 quart
4 quarts	1 gallon			

Measures of mass- Apothecaries

20 grain	1 scruple		3 scruple	1 drachum
8 drachum	1 ounce		12 ounces	1 pound

House hold Measures

1 drop	1 minim	0.04 ml
1 teaspoonful	1 fl.dr.	5 ml
1 dessertspoonful	2 fl.dr.	8 ml
1 tablespoonful	4 fl.dr.	15 ml
1 wineglassful	2 fl.oz.	60 ml
1 teacupful	4 fl.oz.	120 ml
1 tumblerful	8 fl.oz.	240 ml

PRESCRIPTION

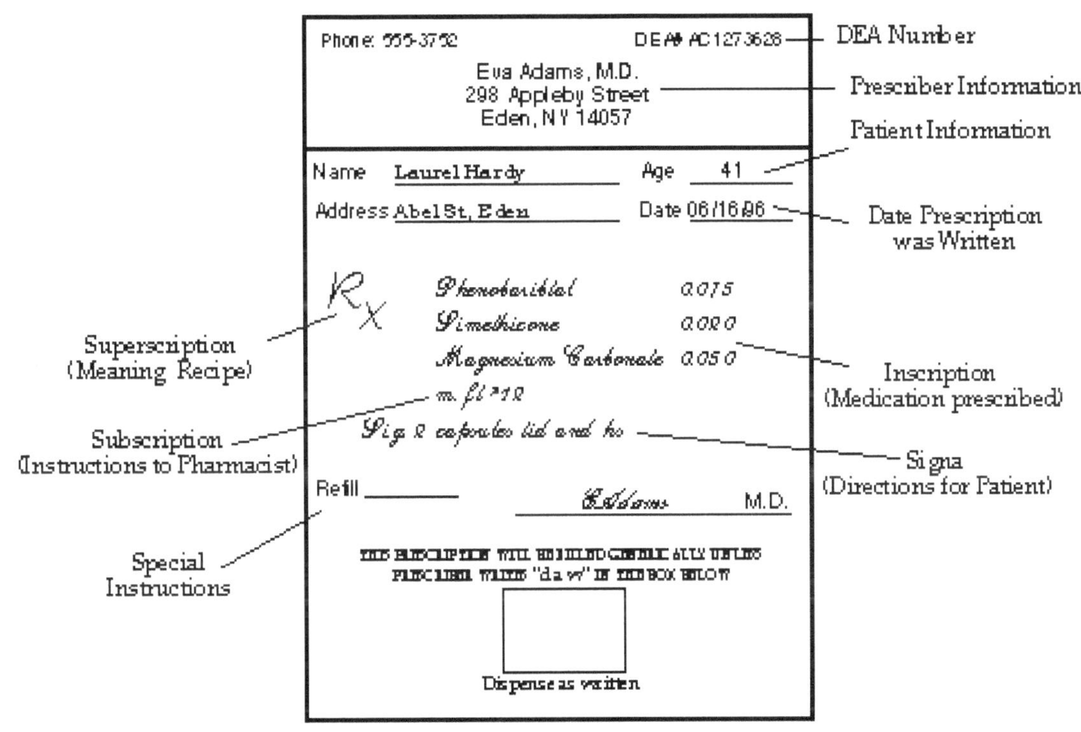

MEDICINE INVOICE

Tin : 12546879				Lic No. : AS124587	

XYZ Medical Hall
New Road, Jalandhar (Pb.)
Tel : 0181-2631089

Invoice No. : 16/12546   Date : 5/03/16
Patient Name : Radhey Shyam   Age : 33   Sex : Male
Prescriber Name : Dr. H. S. Singh, Jalandhar

Sr. No.	Batch No./Exp.	Description	Rate	Quantity	Amount
01	A-145/06-17	Tab. Medigen	200/10	10	200.00
02	CD-91/05-20	Cap. Hygineloic	50/10	5	025.00
03	195/03-18	Inj. Rudoxtrose	35/1	2	070.00
Total : Two Hundred and Ninety Five Rupees Only					295.00

Signature of Pharmacist

GLASS–WARES USED IN PHARMACEUTICS LAB.

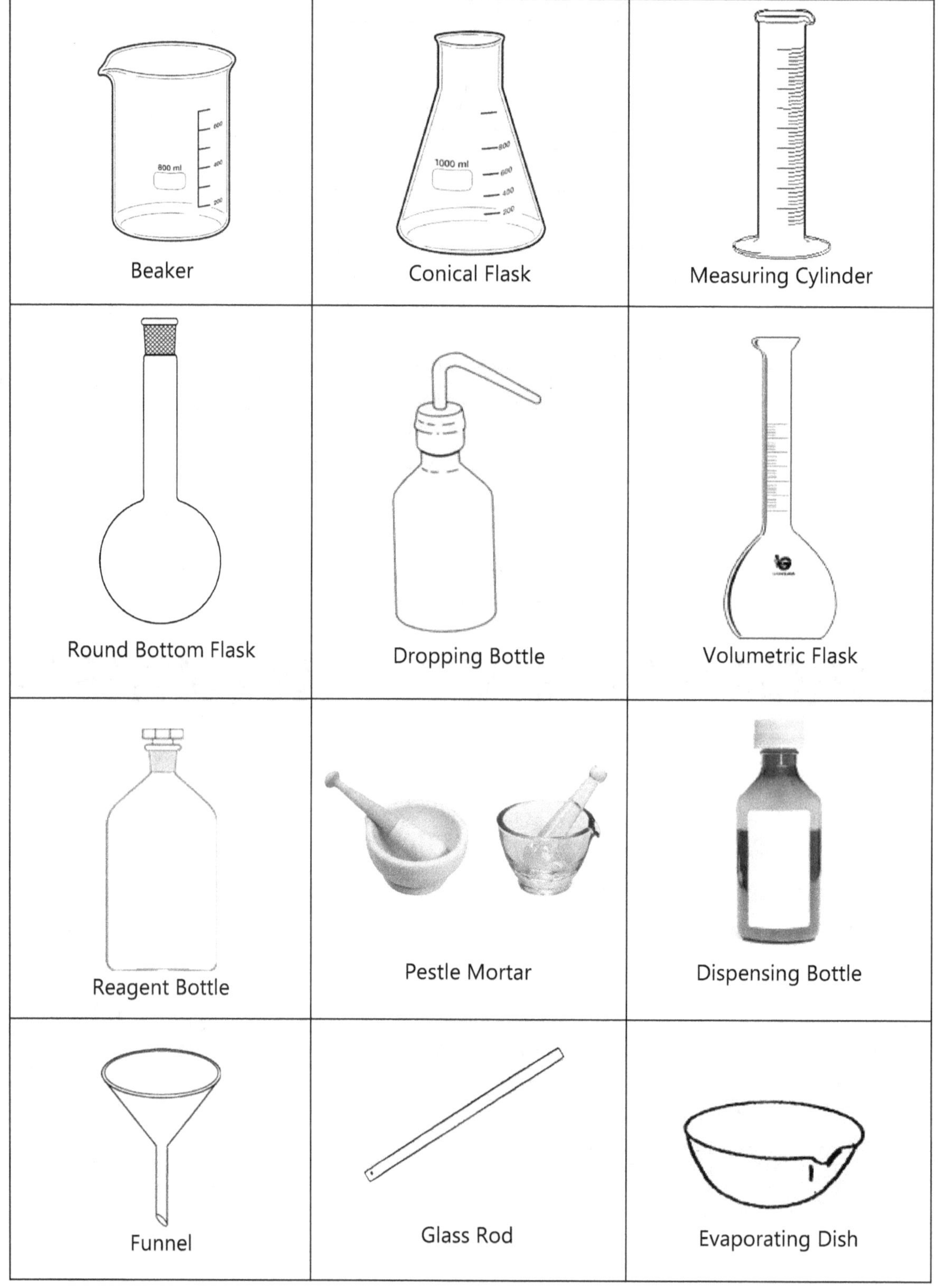

INSTRUMENTS USED IN PHARMACEUTICS LAB.

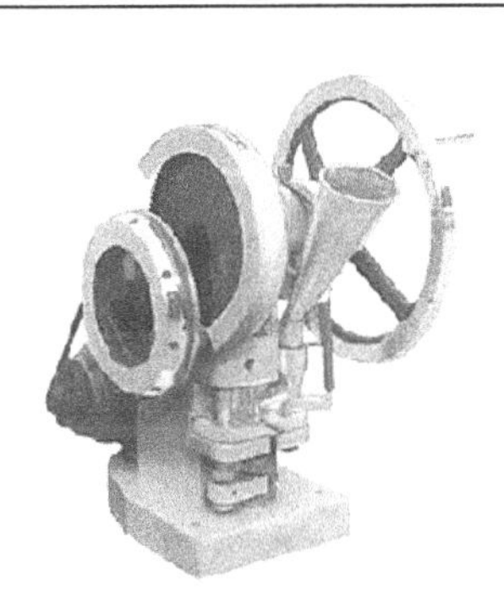

Tablet Compression Machine

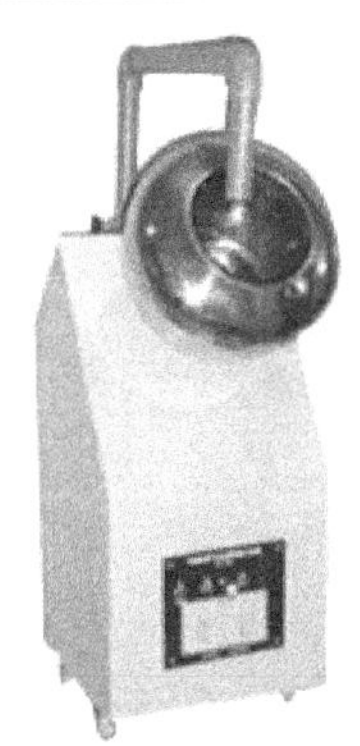

Tablet Coating Machine

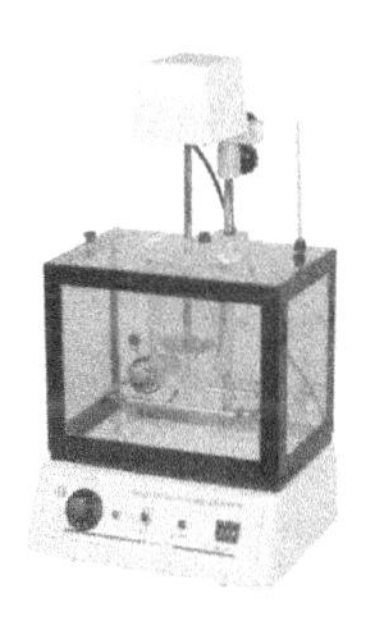

Dissolution Test Apparatus

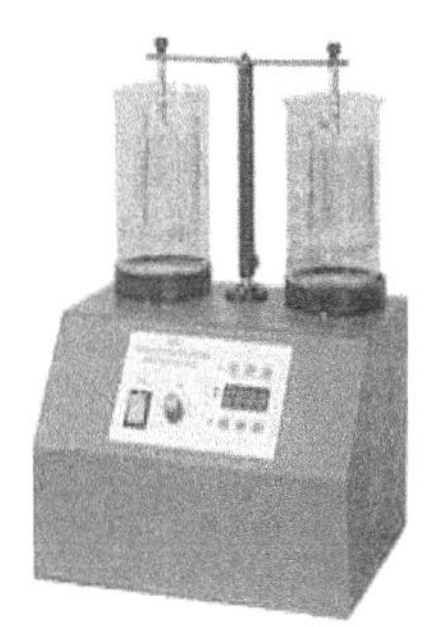

Disintegration Test Apparatus

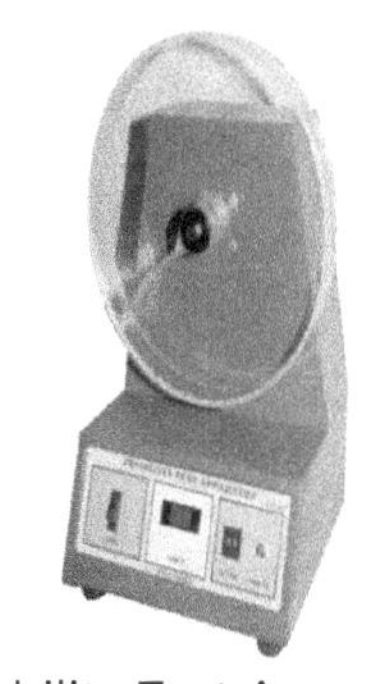

Friability Test Apparatus

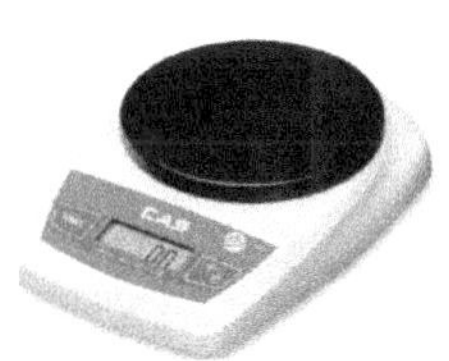

Digital Weighing Machine

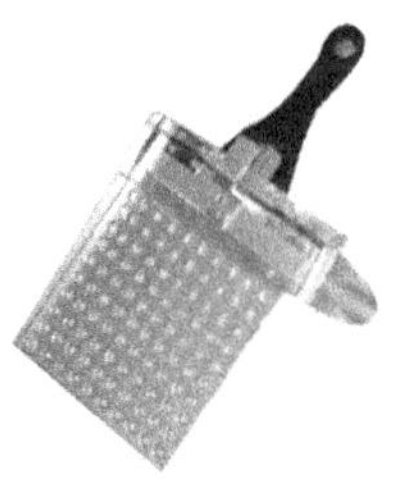

Tablet Counter

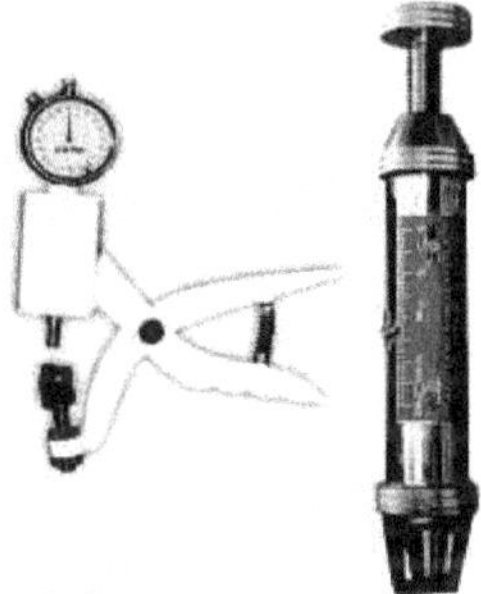

Hardness Tester

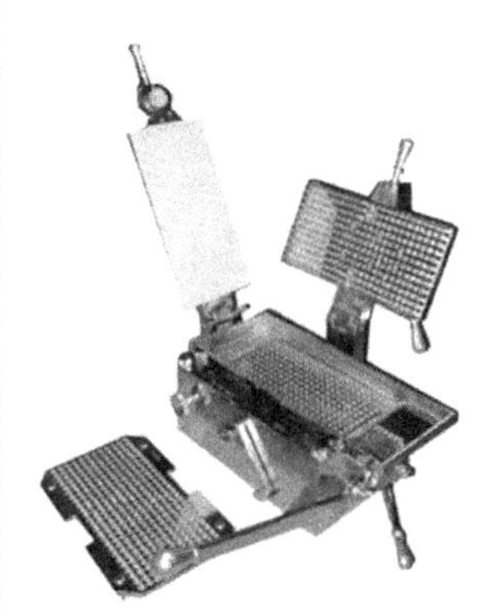

Capsule Filling Machine

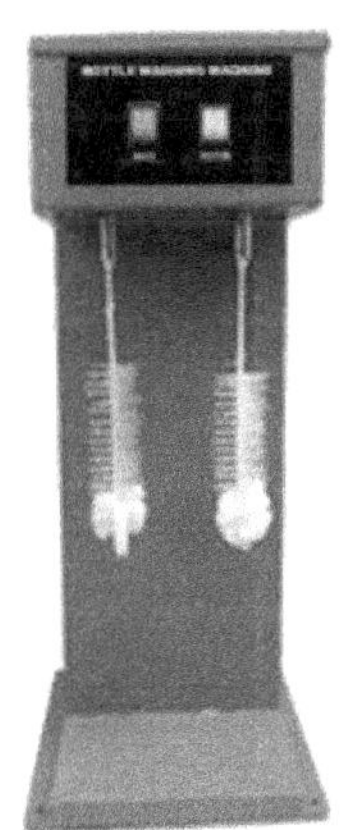

Bottle Washing Machine

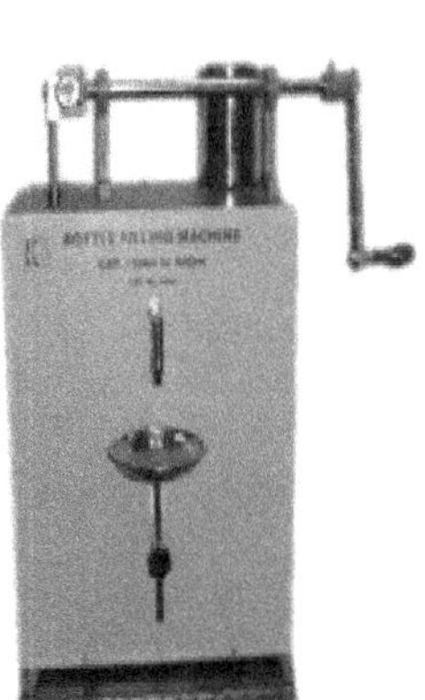

Bottle Filling Machine

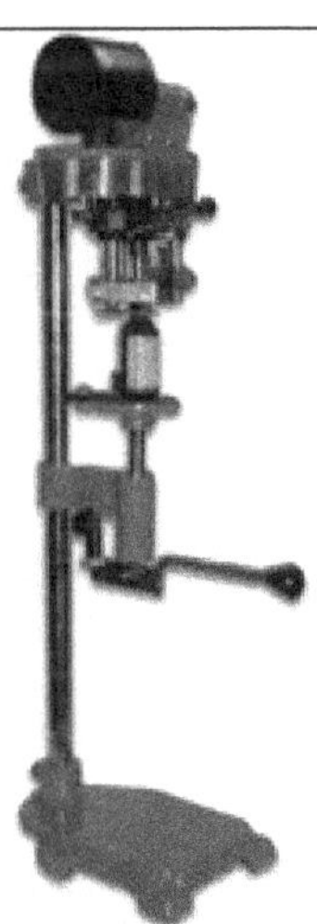

Bottle Sealing Machine

INSTRUMENTS USED IN PHARMACEUTICS LAB.

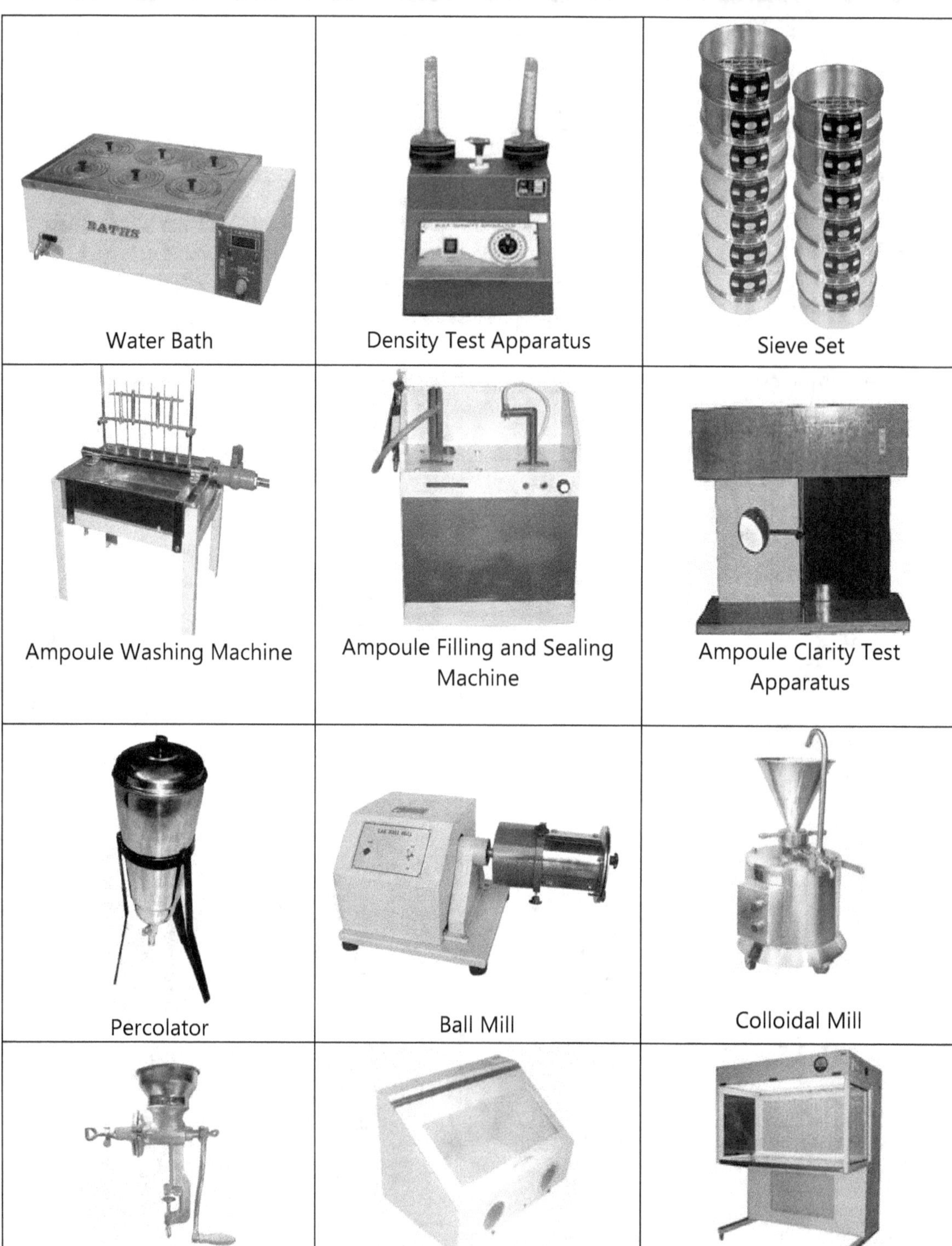

Index ...

Total marks obtained .... out of 1000   **Sign of Subject Teacher**

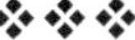

Formulation Table:

Ingredients	Quantity required for 100 ml	Quantity required for _____ ml
Castor oil	25 ml	_______ ml
Water QS	100 ml	______ ml

Calculations:

Castor oil required to prepare 100 ml of mixture = 25 ml

So, for preparation of _____ ml mixture, Castor oil required $= \dfrac{25}{100} \times$ _____ = _____ ml

Label of Preparation:

CASTOR OIL MIXTURE			
Each 100 ml contains Castor oil : 25 ml Water QS : 100.0 ml			
Patient name:		**Age:**	
Sex:		**Weight:**	
Dose: As directed by the physician.			
Mfg. date:		**Exp. Date:**	
Batch no.:		**Price:**	
Prepared by:			

Date :___________   Marks : _________/10

EXPERIMENT NO. 1

- **Aim:** To prepare _________ ml castor oil mixture.
- **Theory:** Physical incompatibility is obtained, when two or more than two substances are combined together, a physical change takes place and an acceptable product is formed. Physical incompatibility occurs due to some of the physical properties of drug and additives such as Immiscibility, Insolubility, Precipitate formation and Liquefaction of solid materials. The physical changes are visible and can be easily corrected by applying the pharmaceutical skill, to obtain a product of uniform dosage, attractive appearance and therapeutic activity.

  In this prescription castor oil is a fixed oil which is immiscible with water. To make the miscible mixture, third emulsifying agent is required to be added, for which gum acacia is most suitable.

  Type of Incompatibility: Physical incompatibility, showing immiscibility.

  Category: Purgative.

  Dose: 15 to 30 ml.

  Uses: Used as purgative.
- **Procedure:** Triturate the gum acacia with small amount of water to make mucilage. To this mucilage add castor oil in small quantity with continuous trituration till a clicking sound is produced. Add more water and triturate it. Transfer this emulsion to the measuring cylinder and add more water to produce required volume.
- **Storage:** Store in a cool place.

VIVA VOCE QUESTIONS

Q.1   What is emulsion?

____

Q.2   Which type of physical incompatibility is present in formulation?

____

Q.3   What is remedy to make the castor oil mixture?

____

❖ ❖ ❖

Formulation Table:

Ingredients	Quantity required for 100 ml	Quantity required for _____ ml
Chalk powder	7 g	_____ g
Tincture of catechu	7 ml	_____ ml
Cinnamon water QS	100 ml	_____ ml

Calculations:

Chalk powder required to prepare 100 ml of mixture = 7.0 g

So, for preparation of _____ ml mixture, Chalk powder required = $\dfrac{7}{100} \times$ _____ = _____ g

Tincture of catechu required to prepare 100 ml of mixture = 7.0 ml

So, for preparation of _____ ml mixture, Tincture required = $\dfrac{7}{100} \times$ _____ = _____ ml

Label of Preparation:

MIXTURE OF CHALK POWDER WITH TINCTURE OF CATECHU			
Each 100 ml contains			
Chalk powder : 7.0 g			
Tincture of catechu : 7.0 ml			
Cinnamon water QS : 100.0 ml			
Patient name:		**Age:**	
Sex:		**Weight:**	
Dose: As directed by the physician.			
Mfg. date:		**Exp. Date:**	
Batch no.:		**Price:**	
Prepared by:			

Date :____________   Marks : __________/10

EXPERIMENT NO. 2

- **Aim:** To prepare _________ ml mixture of chalk powder with tincture of catechu.
- **Theory:** Physical incompatibility is obtained, when two or more than two substances are combined together, a physical change takes place and an acceptable product is formed. Physical incompatibility occurs due to some of the physical properties of drug and additives such as Immiscibility, Insolubility, Precipitate formation and Liquefaction of solid materials. The physical changes are visible and can be easily corrected by applying the pharmaceutical skill, to obtain a product of uniform dosage, attractive appearance and therapeutic activity.

  Type of Incompatibility: Physical incompatibility, showing insolubility.

  Category: Astringent.

  Dose: 15 to 30 ml.

  Uses: Used as antacid.

- **Procedure:** Weigh accurately chalk powder and transfer to a mortar. To this powder, add calculated quantity of compound tragacanth powder and mix thoroughly. Measure $3/4^{th}$ of final volume of cinnamon water, add a small portion to mortar and triturate to form smooth cream. Add tincture of catechu into the centre of the cream with continuous trituration, transfer it to a measuring cylinder and adjust the final volume with cinnamon water.

- **Storage:** Store in a cool place.

VIVA VOCE QUESTIONS

Q.1   What is incompatibility?

____

Q.2   What is physical incompatibility?

____

Q.3   Which type of physical incompatibility is present in formulation?

____

❖❖❖

Formulation Table:

Ingredients	Quantity required for 100 ml	Quantity required for ———— ml
Magnesium carbonate	2 g	———— g
Sodium bicarbonate	2 g	———— g
Citric acid	2 g	———— g
Purified water QS	100 ml	———— ml

Calculations:

Magnesium carbonate required to prepare 100 ml of mixture = 2.0 g

So, for preparation of ___ ml mixture, Magnesium carbonate required = $\dfrac{2}{100} \times$ —— = —— g

Sodium bicarbonate required to prepare 100 ml of mixture = 2.0 g

So, for preparation of _____ ml mixture, Sodium bicarbonate required = $\dfrac{2}{100} \times$ —— = —— g

Citric acid required to prepare 100 ml of mixture = 2.0 g

So, for preparation of _____ ml mixture, Citric acid required = $\dfrac{2}{100} \times$ —— = —— g

Label of Preparation:

MIXTURE OF MAGNESIUM CARBONATE, SODIUM BICARBONATE AND CITRIC ACID			
Each 100 ml contains			
Magnesium carbonate : 2.0 g			
Sodium bicarbonate : 2.0 g			
Citric acid : 2.0 g			
Purified water QS : 100.0 ml			
Patient name:		**Age:**	
Sex:		**Weight:**	
Dose: As directed by the physician.			
Mfg. date:		**Exp. Date:**	
Batch no.:		**Price:**	
Prepared by:			

Date :___________   Marks : _________/10

EXPERIMENT NO. 3

- **Aim:** To prepare _________ ml mixture of magnesium carbonate, sodium bicarbonate and citric acid.
- **Theory:** Physical incompatibility is obtained, when two or more than two substances are combined together, a physical change takes place and an acceptable product is formed. Physical incompatibility occurs due to some of the physical properties of drug and additives such as Immiscibility, Insolubility, Precipitate formation and Liquefaction of solid materials. The physical changes are visible and can be easily corrected by applying the pharmaceutical skill, to obtain a product of uniform dosage, attractive appearance and therapeutic activity.

  Type of Incompatibility: Physical incompatibility, showing insolubility.

  Category: Antacid.

  Dose: 10 to 20 ml.

  Uses: Used as antacid.
- **Procedure:** Weigh separately magnesium carbonate, sodium bicarbonate and citric acid. Take magnesium carbonate in mortar and half the quantity of water with trituration, until a smooth suspension is formed. Dissolve citric acid in a small portion of water, add to the above suspension and let the effervescent ceases completely. Filter the solution if any foreign particles present. Dissolve sodium bicarbonate in a small portion of water by stirring. Mix the above two solutions and let the effervescence ceases completely. Transfer the solution to a measuring cylinder and make up the final volume with water.
- **Storage:** Store in a cool place.

VIVA VOCE QUESTIONS

Q.1   What is incompatibility?

____

Q.2   What is physical incompatibility?

____

Q.3   Which type of physical incompatibility is present in formulation?

____

❖ ❖ ❖

Formulation Table:

Ingredients	Quantity required for 100 g	Quantity required for ______ g
Camphor	34 g	______ g
Menthol	17 g	______ g
Kaolin	49 g	______ g

Calculations:

Camphor required to prepare 100 g of powder = 34 g

So, for preparation of ______ g powder, Camphor required = $\dfrac{34}{100} \times$ ————— = ————— g

Menthol required to prepare 100 g of powder = 17 g

So, for preparation of ______ g powder, Menthol required = $\dfrac{17}{100} \times$ ————— = ————— g

Kaolin required to prepare 100 g of powder = 49 g

So, for preparation of ______ g powder, Kaolin required = $\dfrac{49}{100} \times$ ————— = ————— g

Label of Preparation:

EUTECTIC POWDER			
Each 100 g contains			
Camphor : 34 g			
Menthol : 17 g			
Kaolin : 49 g			
Patient name:		**Age:**	
Sex:		**Weight:**	
Dose: As directed by the physician.			
Mfg. date:		**Exp. Date:**	
Batch no.:		**Price:**	
Prepared by:			

Date : ____________   Marks : ________/10

EXPERIMENT NO. 4

- **Aim:** To prepare ________ g eutectic powder.
- **Theory:** Eutectic means easy melting. When two or more low melting point substances are mixed together, they liquefy due to the formation of a new compound which has a lower melting point, than room temperature. Such substances are called the eutectic substances. This eutectic powder contains camphor and menthol. Each of them acts as an impurity to each other, when they are mixed together. Due to the lower melting point, powder is converted into liquid or semisolid. To overcome this problem kaolin is used as adsorbent, which makes the eutectic mixture dry and free flowing. In this case, eutectic powder is prepared by mixing camphor and menthol with equal quantities of kaolin separately and then both are combined together on a sheet of paper, by light spatulation method.

  Type of Incompatibility: Physical incompatibility, showing liquefaction on mixing.

  Category: Carminative.

  Dose: 1-2 g.

  Uses: Used as carminative.
- **Procedure:** Weigh separately camphor, menthol and kaolin. Dissolve camphor in small quantity of alcohol and allow the alcohol to evaporate at room temperature. After evaporation of alcohol, camphor gets precipitated as fine powder. Mix this fine powder of camphor with half of the portion of kaolin by light spatulation separately. Mix menthol with remaining half of the portion of kaolin by spatulation separately. Mix the above two powder blends uniformly with the help of spatula on a sheet of butter paper. Weigh the prescribed amount of powder and enclose in a double wrapper, lined with butter paper.
- **Storage:** Store in a cool place.

VIVA VOCE QUESTIONS

Q.1   What is eutectic mixture?

____

Q.2   Give examples of eutectic substances.

____

Q.3   How will you dispense eutectic mixture?

____

❖ ❖ ❖

Formulation Table:

Ingredients	Quantity required for 100 ml	Quantity required for ———— ml
Strychnine HCl solution	6 ml	______ ml
Aromatic spirit of ammonia	4 ml	______ ml
Water QS	100 ml	______ ml

Calculations:

Strychnine HCl solution required to prepare 100 ml of powder = 6 ml

So, for preparation of ______ ml mixture, Strychnine HCl solution required

$$= \frac{6}{100} \times \text{————} = \text{————} \; ml$$

Aromatic spirit of ammonia required to prepare 100 ml of mixture = 4 ml

So, for preparation of ______ ml mixture, Aromatic spirit of ammonia required

$$= \frac{4}{100} \times \text{————} = \text{————} \; ml$$

Label of Preparation:

MIXTURE OF ALKALOID SALT WITH ALKALINE SUBSTANCE			
Each 100 ml contains			
Strychnine HCl solution	:	6 ml	
Aromatic spirit of ammonia	:	4 ml	
Water QS	:	100 ml	
Patient name:		**Age:**	
Sex:		**Weight:**	
Dose: As directed by the physician.			
Mfg. date:		**Exp. Date:**	
Batch no.:		**Price:**	
Prepared by:			

Date :__________   Marks : ________/10

EXPERIMENT NO. 5

- **Aim:** To prepare ________ ml mixture of alkaloid salt with alkaline substance.
- **Theory:** This formulation shows tolerated type chemical incompatibility; because strychnine HCl is an alkaloidal salt, but aromatic spirit of ammonia is an alkaline substance. When they react together, precipitate of strychnine will be formed because the quantity of strychnine HCl prescribed is much more than its solubility. Aromatic spirit of ammonia contains alcohol, which is in negligible quantity to dissolve the precipitated strychnine.

  Type of Incompatibility: Chemical incompatibility, showing precipitation.

  Category: Stimulant.

  Dose: 4 to 5 ml.

  Uses: Used as CNS stimulant.

- **Procedure:** Divide the purified water into two equal portions. Mix strychnine HCl solution in one portion of water. Mix aromatic spirit of ammonia with little quantity of water. Mix both the solutions slowly by continuous stirring. Transfer the solution to a measuring cylinder and make up the final volume with water.

- **Storage:** Store in a cool place.

VIVA VOCE QUESTIONS

Q.1   What is chemical incompatibility?

____

Q.2   Which type of incompatibility is present in the formulation?

____

Q.3   Explain the remedy used in the preparation of the formulation?

____

❖ ❖ ❖

Formulation Table:

Ingredients	Quantity required for 100 ml	Quantity required for ——— ml
Quinine hydrochloride	1.25 g	_____ g
Sodium salicylate	4 g	_____ g
Water QS	100 ml	_____ ml

Calculations:

Quinine hydrochloride required to prepare 100 ml of mixture = 1.25 g

So, for preparation of _______ ml mixture, Quinine hydrochloride required

$$= \frac{1.25}{100} \times \text{——} = \text{——} \, g$$

Sodium salicylate required to prepare 100 ml of mixture = 4 g

So, for preparation of _______ ml mixture, Sodium salicylate required

$$= \frac{4}{100} \times \text{——} = \text{——} \, g$$

Label of Preparation:

MIXTURE OF QUININE AND SODIUM SALICYLATE			
Each 100 ml contains			
Quinine hydrochloride : 1.25 g			
Sodium salicylate : 4 g			
Water QS : 100 ml			
Patient name:		**Age:**	
Sex:		**Weight:**	
Dose: As directed by the physician.			
Mfg. date:		**Exp. Date:**	
Batch no.:		**Price:**	
Prepared by:			

Date :___________   Marks : _________/10

EXPERIMENT NO. 6

- **Aim:** To prepare _________ ml mixture of quinine and sodium salicylate.
- **Theory:** This prescription shows chemical incompatibility because quinine hydrochloride is an alkaloidal salt, which when reacts with sodium salicylate, it will be precipitated out as quinine salicylate. The precipitate is indiffusible in nature. This indiffusible precipitate is diffused with the help of suspending agent tragacanth.

  Type of Incompatibility: Chemical incompatibility, showing precipitation.

  Category: Analgesic.

  Dose: 4 to 5 ml.

  Uses: Used in treatment of malarial fever.

- **Procedure:** Weigh separately sodium salicylate and compound powder of tragacanth and transfer into mortar. Triturate them to mix properly. Weigh accurately quinine hydrochloride and dissolve in the little quantity of water. Add this solution into the mortar. Mix well by trituration. Transfer the above mixture into measuring cylinder. Rinse the pestle and mortar with water and then transfer to the measuring cylinder. Adjust the final volume with water and mix well.
- **Storage:** Store in a cool place.

VIVA VOCE QUESTIONS

Q.1   What is chemical incompatibility?

____

Q.2   Which type of incompatibility is present in the formulation?

____

Q.3   Explain the remedy used in the preparation of the formulation?

____

❖ ❖ ❖

Formulation Table:

Ingredients	Quantity required for 100 ml	Quantity required for ——— ml
Sodium salicylate	4.5 g	_____ g
Simple syrup	23 ml	_____ ml
Tincture of lemon	1.5 ml	_____ ml
Water QS	100 ml	_____ ml

Calculations:

Sodium salicylate required to prepare 100 ml of mixture = 4.5 g

So, for preparation of _____ ml mixture, Sodium salicylate required $= \dfrac{4.5}{100} \times$ —— = —— g

Simple syrup required to prepare 100 ml of mixture = 23 ml

So, for preparation of _____ ml mixture, Simple syrup required $= \dfrac{23}{100} \times$ —— = —— ml

Tincture of lemon required to prepare 100 ml of mixture = 1.5 ml

So, for preparation of _____ ml mixture, Tincture of lemon required $= \dfrac{1.5}{100} \times$ —— = —— ml

Label of Preparation:

MIXTURE OF SOLUBLE SALICYLATE WITH ACID			
Each 100 ml contains			
Sodium salicylate : 4.5 ml			
Simple syrup : 23 ml			
Tincture of lemon : 1.5 ml			
Water QS : 100 ml			
Patient name:		**Age:**	
Sex:		**Weight:**	
Dose: As directed by the physician.			
Mfg. date:		**Exp. Date:**	
Batch no.:		**Price:**	
Prepared by:			

Date :___________   Marks :________/10

EXPERIMENT NO. 7

- **Aim:** To prepare _______ ml mixture of soluble salicylate with acid.
- **Theory:** This prescription shows the adjusted type chemical incompatibility due to the acid-base reaction between lemon syrup and sodium salicylate. Lemon syrup contains citric acid. Due to its strong acidic nature, it decomposes sodium salicylate into salicylic acid. The lemon syrup is adjusted by the simple syrup and tincture of lemon is added as the flavouring agent.

  Type of Incompatibility: Chemical incompatibility, showing precipitation.

  Category: Analgesic.

  Dose: 4 to 5 ml.

  Uses: Used to get relief in pain.
- **Procedure:** Accurately weigh required quantity of sodium salicylate and dissolve it in 75% quantity of water in a beaker. Filter the solution through a muslin cloth, directly to previously tare amber coloured bottle. To the filtrate add measured quantity of simple syrup and tincture of lemon. Mix well and adjust the final volume with remaining amount of water.
- **Storage:** Store in a cool place.

VIVA VOCE QUESTIONS

Q.1   What is adjusted chemical incompatibility?

____

Q.2   Which type of incompatibility is present in the formulation?

____

Q.3   Explain the remedy used in the preparation of the formulation?

____

❖❖❖

Formulation Table:

Ingredients	Quantity required for 100 ml	Quantity required for —— ml
Sodium salicylate	2.0 g	—— g
Ferric chloride solution	0.5 ml	—— ml
Sodium bicarbonate	4.0 g	—— g
Water QS	100 ml	—— ml

Calculations:

Sodium salicylate required to prepare 100 ml of mixture = 2.0 g

So, for preparation of ____ ml mixture, Sodium salicylate required $= \dfrac{2.0}{100} \times$ —— = —— g

Ferric chloride solution required to prepare 100 ml of mixture = 0.5 ml

So, for preparation of __ ml mixture, Ferric chloride solution required $= \dfrac{0.5}{100} \times$ — = — ml

Sodium bicarbonate required to prepare 100 ml of mixture = 4.0 g

So, for preparation of ____ ml mixture, Sodium bicarbonate required $= \dfrac{4.0}{100} \times$ — = — g

Label of Preparation:

MIXTURE OF SALICYLATE AND FERRIC SALT			
Each 100 ml contains Sodium salicylate : 2.0 g Ferric chloride solution : 0.5 ml Sodium bicarbonate : 4.0 g Water QS : 100 ml			
Patient name:		**Age:**	
Sex:		**Weight:**	
Dose: As directed by the physician.			
Mfg. date:		**Exp. Date:**	
Batch no.:		**Price:**	
Prepared by:			

Date :______________   Marks : _________/10

EXPERIMENT NO. 8

- **Aim:** To prepare _________ ml mixture of salicylate and ferric salt.
- **Theory:** This prescription shows the adjusted type chemical incompatibility due to the acid-base reaction between ferric chloride and sodium salicylate. The ferric salicylate will be predicated out which is violet in colour and also insoluble and indiffusible in water. In this prescription precipitated ferric salicylate easily dissolves in sodium bicarbonate solution.

  Type of Incompatibility: Chemical incompatibility, showing precipitation.

  Category: Astringent.

  Dose: 4 to 5 ml.

  Uses: Used in anaemia as a supplement during haemorrhage.

- **Procedure:** Accurately weigh required quantity of sodium salicylate and sodium bicarbonate. Dissolve it in 75% quantity of water in a beaker. Separately prepare ferric chloride solution in water. Mix the above solution and ferric chloride solution with continuous stirring and allow elaborating the entire carbon dioxide gas completely. Filter the solution through the muslin cloth and transfer the filtrate to a measuring cylinder. Adjust the final volume with purified water.
- **Storage:** Store in a cool place.

VIVA VOCE QUESTIONS

Q.1   What is adjusted chemical incompatibility?

____

Q.2   Which type of incompatibility is present in the formulation?

____

Q.3   Explain the remedy used in the preparation of the formulation?

____

❖ ❖ ❖

Formulation Table:

Ingredients	Quantity required for 15 g	Quantity required for —— g
POWDER - A		
Sodium potassium tartrate	7.5 g	—— g
Sodium bicarbonate	2.5 g	—— g
POWDER - B		
Tartaric acid	5.0 g	—— g

Calculations:

Sodium potassium tartrate required to prepare 15 g of powder = 7.5 g

So, for preparation of __ g powder, Sodium potassium tartrate required = $\dfrac{7.5}{15} \times$ —— = —— g

Sodium bicarbonate required to prepare 15 g of powder = 2.5 g

So, for preparation of _____ g powder, Sodium bicarbonate required = $\dfrac{2.5}{15} \times$ —— = —— g

Tartaric acid required to prepare 15 g of powder = 5 g

So, for preparation of _____ g powder, tartaric acid required = $\dfrac{5}{15} \times$ —— = —— g

Label of Preparation:

SEIDLIZ DIVIDED POWDER			
Each 15 g contains Sodium potassium tartrate : 7.5 g Sodium bicarbonate : 2.5 g Tartaric acid : 5.0 g			
Patient name:		**Age:**	
Sex:		**Weight:**	
Dose: As directed by the physician.			
Mfg. date:		**Exp. Date:**	
Batch no.:		**Price:**	
Prepared by:			

Date : _____________   Marks : _________/10

EXPERIMENT NO. 9

- **Aim:** To prepare _________ g seidliz divided powder.

- **Theory:** Pharmaceutical powders are mixture of finely divided drugs or chemicals in dry forms. They are intended for internal or external use for many diseases. Pharmaceutical powders may be classified on the basis of dispensing of powders. These are bulk powder for external use, bulk powder for internal use, divided powder for internal use, effervescent powder or granules.

  The effervescent powder consists of two powders as given in formula. The powder A are dissolved in water, then Powder B are added. The mixture is stirred and the product is taken while effervescing.

  Category: Effervescent powder.

  Dose: One pair of powders.

  Uses: Effervescent draught.

- **Procedure:** Mix sodium potassium tartrate and sodium bicarbonate uniformly. Similarly powder tartaric acid separately. Double wrap both powders using an inner wrapper of wax paper. Wrap both powders in different colour papers. Pack in pairs should consist of powders A and B.

- **Storage:** Store in a low humidity and light place.

VIVA VOCE QUESTIONS

Q.1   What is the effervescent powder?

____

Q.2   Why both powders are packed separately?

____

Q.3   How to take this powder?

____

❖ ❖ ❖

Formulation Table:

Ingredients	Quantity required for 200 g	Quantity required for _____ g
Chalk powder	15 g	_____ g
Cinnamon powder	60 g	_____ g
Nutmeg powder	48 g	_____ g
Clove powder	24 g	_____ g
Cardamom powder	18 g	_____ g
Sucrose	35 g	_____ g

Calculations:

Chalk powder required to prepare 200 g of powder = 15 g

So, for preparation of _____ g powder, Chalk powder required $= \dfrac{15}{200} \times$ ————— = ————— g

Cinnamon powder required to prepare 200 g of powder = 60 g

So, for preparation of _____ g powder, Cinnamon powder required $= \dfrac{60}{200} \times$ ————— = ————— g

Nutmeg powder required to prepare 200 g of powder = 48 g

So, for preparation of _____ g powder, Nutmeg powder required $= \dfrac{48}{200} \times$ ————— = ————— g

Clove powder required to prepare 200 g of powder = 24 g

So, for preparation of _____ g powder, Clove powder required $= \dfrac{24}{200} \times$ ————— = ————— g

Cardamom powder required to prepare 200 g of powder = 18 g

So, for preparation of _____ g powder, Cardamom powder required $= \dfrac{18}{200} \times$ ————— = ————— g

Sucrose required to prepare 200 g of powder = 35 g

So, for preparation of _____ g powder, sucrose required $= \dfrac{35}{200} \times$ ————— = ————— g

Label of Preparation:

AROMATIC CHALK POWDER			
Each 200 g contains			
Chalk powder	: 15 g		
Cinnamon powder	: 60 g		
Nutmeg powder	: 48 g		
Clove powder	: 24 g		
Cardamom powder	: 18 g		
Sucrose	: 35 g		
Patient name:		**Age:**	
Sex:		**Weight:**	
Dose: As directed by the physician.			
Mfg. date:		**Exp. Date:**	
Batch no.:		**Price:**	
Prepared by:			

Date : _____________   Marks : _________/10

EXPERIMENT NO. 10

- **Aim:** To prepare _________ g Aromatic chalk powder.

- **Theory:** Pharmaceutical powders are mixture of finely divided drugs or chemicals in dry forms. They are intended for internal or external use for many diseases. Pharmaceutical powders may be classified on the basis of dispensing of powders. These are bulk powder for external use, bulk powder for internal use, divided powder for internal use, effervescent powder or granules.

  Uses: Carminative and antacid.

  Dose: As directed by physician.

- **Procedure:** Mix all the ingredients in ascending order of their weight and triturate uniformly. Pass through suitable sieve and preserve in a well-closed container.

- **Storage:** Store in an air-tight container.

VIVA VOCE QUESTIONS

Q.1   What is the compound powder?

____

Q.2   What is the use of chalk?

____

Q.3   What is carminative?

____

❖ ❖ ❖

Formulation Table:

Ingredients	Quantity required for 2 g	Quantity required for _____ g
Magnesium trisilicate	0.25 g	_____ g
Chalk powder	0.25 g	_____ g
Heavy magnesium carbonate	0.25 g	_____ g
Sodium bicarbonate	0.25 g	_____ g

Calculations:

Magnesium trisilicate required to prepare 2.0 g of powder = 0.25 g

So, for preparation of _____ g powder, Magnesium trisilicate required = $\dfrac{0.25}{2.0}$ × —— = —— g

Chalk powder required to prepare 2.0 g of powder = 0.25 g

So, for preparation of _____ g powder, Chalk powder required = $\dfrac{0.25}{2.0}$ × —— = —— g

Heavy magnesium carbonate required to prepare 2.0 g of powder = 0.25 g

So, for preparation of _____ g powder, Heavy magnesium carbonate required = $\dfrac{0.25}{2.0}$ × — = — g

Sodium bicarbonate required to prepare 2.0 g of powder = 0.25 g

So, for preparation of _____ g powder, Sodium bicarbonate required = $\dfrac{0.25}{2.0}$ × —— = —— g

Label of Preparation:

COMPOUND MAGNESIUM TRISILICATE ORAL POWDER			
Each 2 g contains			
Magnesium trisilicate	: 0.25 g		
Chalk powder	: 0.25 g		
Heavy magnesium carbonate	: 0.25 g		
Sodium bicarbonate	: 0.25 g		
Patient name:		**Age:**	
Sex:		**Weight:**	
Dose: As directed by the physician.			
Mfg. date:		**Exp. Date:**	
Batch no.:		**Price:**	
Prepared by:			

Date :___________   Marks : ________/10

EXPERIMENT NO. 11

- **Aim:** To prepare _________ g compound magnesium trisilicate oral powder.
- **Theory:** Pharmaceutical powders are mixture of finely divided drugs or chemicals in dry forms. They are intended for internal or external use for many diseases. Pharmaceutical powders may be classified on the basis of dispensing of powders. These are bulk powder for external use, bulk powder for internal use, divided powder for internal use, effervescent powder or granules.

  Uses: Antacid.

  Dose: 0.3 to 2.0 g.

- **Procedure:** Mix all the ingredients in ascending order of their weight and triturate uniformly. Pass through suitable sieve and preserve in a well-closed container.
- **Storage:** Store in an air-tight container.

VIVA VOCE QUESTIONS

Q.1   Why magnesium trisilicate oral powder is prepared?

____

Q.2   What is antacid?

____

Q.3   What is the use of magnesium carbonate?

____

❖❖❖

Formulation Table:

Ingredients	Quantity required for 2 g	Quantity required for ______ g
Light kaolin	1.0 g	______ g
Heavy magnesium carbonate	0.67 g	______ g
Sodium bicarbonate	0.33 g	______ g

Calculations:

Light kaolin required to prepare 2.0 g of powder = 1.0 g

So, for preparation of ______ g powder, Light kaolin required $= \dfrac{1}{2.0} \times \text{------} = \text{------} \ g$

Heavy magnesium carbonate required to prepare 2.0 g of powder = 0.67 g

So, for preparation of ______ g powder, Heavy magnesium carbonate required

$$= \dfrac{0.67}{2.0} \times \text{------} = \text{------} \ g$$

Sodium bicarbonate required to prepare 2.0 g of powder = 0.33 g

So, for preparation of ______ g powder, Sodium bicarbonate required

$$= \dfrac{0.33}{2.0} \times \text{------} = \text{------} \ g$$

Label of Preparation:

KAOLIN COMPOUND POWDER			
Each 2 g contains			
Magnesium trisilicate	:	1.0 g	
Heavy magnesium carbonate	:	0.67 g	
Sodium bicarbonate	:	0.33 g	
Patient name:		**Age:**	
Sex:		**Weight:**	
Dose: As directed by the physician.			
Mfg. date:		**Exp. Date:**	
Batch no.:		**Price:**	
Prepared by:			

Date :___________ Marks : _________/10

EXPERIMENT NO. 12

- **Aim:** To prepare _________ g kaolin compound powder.

- **Theory:** Pharmaceutical powders are mixture of finely divided drugs or chemicals in dry forms. They are intended for internal or external use for many diseases. Pharmaceutical powders may be classified on the basis of dispensing of powders. These are bulk powder for external use, bulk powder for internal use, divided powder for internal use, effervescent powder or granules.

  Uses: Diarrhoea.

  Dose: As directed by physician.

- **Procedure:** Mix all the ingredients in ascending order of their weight and triturate uniformly. Pass through suitable sieve and preserve in a well-closed container.

- **Storage:** Store in an air-tight container.

VIVA VOCE QUESTIONS

Q.1   What is light kaolin?

____

Q.2   What is diarrhoea?

____

Q.3   What is the method of preparation?

____

❖ ❖ ❖

Formulation Table:

Ingredients	Quantity required for 10 g	Quantity required for _____ g
Magnesium oxide	0.50 g	_____ g
Starch in powder	1.5 g	_____ g
Purified talc	8.0 g	_____ g

Calculations:

Magnesium oxide required to prepare 10 g of powder = 0.50 g

So, for preparation of _____ g powder, Magnesium oxide required = $\dfrac{0.50}{10.0} \times$ ——— = ——— g

Starch required to prepare 10 g of powder = 1.5 g

So, for preparation of _____ g powder, Starch required = $\dfrac{1.5}{10.0} \times$ ——— = ——— g

Purified talc required to prepare 10 g of powder = 8.0 g

So, for preparation of _____ g powder, Purified talc required = $\dfrac{8.0}{10.0} \times$ ——— = ——— g

Label of Preparation:

<table>
<tr><th colspan="4">TALC DUSTING POWDER</th></tr>
<tr><td colspan="4">Each 10 g contains</td></tr>
<tr><td colspan="4">Magnesium oxide : 0.50 g</td></tr>
<tr><td colspan="4">Starch in powder : 1.5 g</td></tr>
<tr><td colspan="4">Purified talc : 8.0 g</td></tr>
<tr><td>Patient name:</td><td></td><td>Age:</td><td></td></tr>
<tr><td>Sex:</td><td></td><td>Weight:</td><td></td></tr>
<tr><td colspan="4">Dose: As directed by the physician.</td></tr>
<tr><td>Mfg. date:</td><td></td><td>Exp. Date:</td><td></td></tr>
<tr><td>Batch no.:</td><td></td><td>Price:</td><td></td></tr>
<tr><td colspan="4">Prepared by:</td></tr>
</table>

Date :___________   Marks : ________/10

EXPERIMENT NO. 13

- **Aim:** To prepare ________ g talc dusting powder.
- **Theory:** Pharmaceutical powders are mixture of finely divided drugs or chemicals in dry forms. They are intended for internal or external use for many diseases. Pharmaceutical powders may be classified on the basis of dispensing of powders. These are bulk powder for external use, bulk powder for internal use, divided powder for internal use, effervescent powder or granules.

  Uses: Pharmaceutical aid, dusting powder.

  Dose: For external use.

- **Procedure:** Mix all the ingredients in ascending order of their weight and triturate uniformly. Pass through suitable sieve and preserve in a well-closed container.
- **Storage:** Store in a well-closed wide-mouthed bottle.

VIVA VOCE QUESTIONS

Q.1   What are dusting powders?

____

Q.2   How dusting powder is prepared?

____

Q.3   Give application of dusting powder?

____

❖ ❖ ❖

Formulation Table:

Ingredients	Quantity required for 10 g	Quantity required for ______ g
Salicylic acid	0.30 g	______ g
Boric acid	0.50 g	______ g
Purified talc	9.2 g	______ g

Calculations:

Salicylic acid required to prepare 10 g of powder = 0.30 g

So, for preparation of ______ g powder, Salicylic acid required = $\dfrac{0.30}{10.0} \times$ —— = —— g

Boric acid required to prepare 10 g of powder = 0.50 g

So, for preparation of ______ g powder, Boric acid required = $\dfrac{0.50}{10.0} \times$ —— = —— g

Purified talc required to prepare 10 g of powder = 9.2 g

So, for preparation of ______ g powder, Purified talc required = $\dfrac{9.2}{10.0} \times$ —— = —— g

Label of Preparation:

SALICYLIC ACID COMPOUND DUSTING POWDER			
Each 10 g contains Salicylic acid : 0.30 g Boric acid : 0.50 g Purified talc : 9.2 g			
Patient name:		**Age:**	
Sex:		**Weight:**	
Dose: As directed by the physician.			
Mfg. date:		**Exp. Date:**	
Batch no.:		**Price:**	
Prepared by:			

Date :___________   Marks : _________/10

EXPERIMENT NO. 14

- **Aim:** To prepare _________ g salicylic acid compound dusting powder.

- **Theory:** Pharmaceutical powders are mixture of finely divided drugs or chemicals in dry forms. They are intended for internal or external use for many diseases. Pharmaceutical powders may be classified on the basis of dispensing of powders. These are bulk powder for external use, bulk powder for internal use, divided powder for internal use, effervescent powder or granules.

  Uses: Germicide, used in local infection on skin.

  Dose: For external use.

- **Procedure:** Mix all the ingredients in ascending order of their weight and triturate uniformly. Pass through suitable sieve and preserve in a well-closed container.

- **Storage:** Store in a well-closed wide-mouthed bottle.

VIVA VOCE QUESTIONS

Q.1   What is the use of boric acid?

____

Q.2   What is the local anti-infective?

____

Q.3   Which type of container is suitable for dusting powders?

____

❖ ❖ ❖

Formulation Table:

Ingredients	Quantity required for 10 g	Quantity required for _____ g
Zinc oxide	5.0 g	_____ g
Starch powder	5.0 g	_____ g

Calculations:

Zinc oxide required to prepare 10 g of powder = 5.0 g

So, for preparation of _____ g powder, Zinc oxide required = $\dfrac{5.0}{10.0} \times$ —— = —— g

Starch powder required to prepare 10 g of powder = 5.0 g

So, for preparation of _____ g powder, Starch powder required = $\dfrac{5.0}{10.0} \times$ —— = —— g

Label of Preparation:

SALICYLIC ACID COMPOUND DUSTING POWDER			
Each 10 g contains			
Zinc oxide : 5.0 g			
Starch powder : 5.0 g			
Patient name:		**Age:**	
Sex:		**Weight:**	
Dose: As directed by the physician.			
Mfg. date:		**Exp. Date:**	
Batch no.:		**Price:**	
Prepared by:			

Date :___________   Marks : _________/10

EXPERIMENT NO. 15

- **Aim:** To prepare _________ g zinc oxide and starch dusting powder.

- **Theory:** Pharmaceutical powders are mixture of finely divided drugs or chemicals in dry forms. They are intended for internal or external use for many diseases. Pharmaceutical powders may be classified on the basis of dispensing of powders. These are bulk powder for external use, bulk powder for internal use, divided powder for internal use, effervescent powder or granules.

  Uses: Astringent, protective and anti-septic.

  Dose: For external use.

- **Procedure:** Mix all the ingredients in ascending order of their weight and triturate uniformly. Pass through suitable sieve and preserve in a well-closed container.

- **Storage:** Store in a well-closed wide-mouthed bottle.

VIVA VOCE QUESTIONS

Q.1   What is antiseptic powder?

____

Q.2   What is astringent?

____

Q.3   Define protective powder.

____

❖ ❖ ❖

Formulation Table:

Ingredients	Quantity required for 10 g	Quantity required for _____ g
Tragacanth powder	1.5 g	_____ g
Acacia powder	2.0 g	_____ g
Starch powder	2.0 g	_____ g
Sucrose powder	4.5 g	_____ g

Calculations:

Tragacanth powder required to prepare 10 g of powder = 1.5 g

So, for preparation of _____ g powder, Tragacanth powder required = $\dfrac{1.5}{10.0} \times \text{—} = \text{—}$ g

Acacia powder required to prepare 10 g of powder = 2.0 g

So, for preparation of _____ g powder, Acacia powder required = $\dfrac{2.0}{10.0} \times \text{———} = \text{———}$ g

Starch powder required to prepare 10 g of powder = 2.0 g

So, for preparation of _____ g powder, Starch powder required = $\dfrac{2.0}{10.0} \times \text{———} = \text{———}$ g

Sucrose powder required to prepare 10 g of powder = 4.5 g

So, for preparation of _____ g powder, Sucrose powder required = $\dfrac{4.5}{10.0} \times \text{———} = \text{———}$ g

Label of Preparation:

COMPOUND TRAGACANTH POWDER			
Each 10 g contains			
Tragacanth powder : 1.5 g			
Acacia powder : 2.0 g			
Starch powder : 2.0 g			
Sucrose powder : 4.5 g			
Patient name:		**Age:**	
Sex:		**Weight:**	
Dose: As directed by the physician.			
Mfg. date:		**Exp. Date:**	
Batch no.:		**Price:**	
Prepared by:			

Date :____________   Marks :________/10

EXPERIMENT NO. 16

- **Aim:** To prepare ________ g compound tragacanth powder.

- **Theory:** Pharmaceutical powders are mixture of finely divided drugs or chemicals in dry forms. They are intended for internal or external use for many diseases. Pharmaceutical powders may be classified on the basis of dispensing of powders. These are bulk powder for external use, bulk powder for internal use, divided powder for internal use, effervescent powder or granules.

  Uses: Pharmaceutical aid.

  Dose: As directed by physician.

- **Procedure:** Mix all the ingredients in ascending order of their weight and triturate uniformly. Pass through suitable sieve and preserve in a well-closed container.

- **Storage:** Store in a well-closed container and protect from atmospheric moisture.

VIVA VOCE QUESTIONS

Q.1   What is the use of tragacanth?

____

Q.2   What is the use of acacia?

____

Q.3   Define pharmaceutical aid powder.

____

❖❖❖

Formulation Table:

Ingredients	Quantity required for 10 g	Quantity required for _____ g
Senna leaf powder	1.6 g	_____ g
Liquorice powder	1.6 g	_____ g
Fennel powder	0.80 g	_____ g
Sulphur powder	0.80 g	_____ g
Sucrose	5.2 g	_____ g

Calculations:

Senna leaf powder required to prepare 10 g of powder = 1.6 g

So, for preparation of _____ g powder, Senna leaf powder required = $\dfrac{1.6}{10.0} \times \text{---} = \text{---}$ g

Liquorice powder quantity same as Senna leaf = _____ g

Fennel powder required to prepare 10 g of powder = 0.8 g

So, for preparation of _____ g powder, Fennel powder required = $\dfrac{0.8}{10.0} \times \text{---} = \text{---}$ g

Sulphur powder quantity same as Fennel powder = _____ g

Sucrose required to prepare 10 g of powder = 5.2 g

So, for preparation of _____ g powder, Sucrose required = $\dfrac{5.2}{10.0} \times \text{---} = \text{---}$ g

Label of Preparation:

LIQUORICE COMPOUND POWDER		
Each 10 g contains		
Senna leaf powder : 1.6 g		
Liquorice powder : 1.6 g		
Fennel powder : 0.80 g		
Sulphur powder : 0.80 g		
Sucrose : 5.2 g		
Patient name:		**Age:**	
Sex:		**Weight:**	
Dose: As directed by the physician.			
Mfg. date:		**Exp. Date:**	
Batch no.:		**Price:**	
Prepared by:			

Date :___________   Marks : ________/10

EXPERIMENT NO. 17

- **Aim:** To prepare ________ g liquorice compound powder.

- **Theory:** Pharmaceutical powders are mixture of finely divided drugs or chemicals in dry forms. They are intended for internal or external use for many diseases. Pharmaceutical powders may be classified on the basis of dispensing of powders. These are bulk powder for external use, bulk powder for internal use, divided powder for internal use, effervescent powder or granules.

  Uses: Laxative.

  Dose: 4 to 8 g.

- **Procedure:** Mix all the ingredients in ascending order of their weight and triturate uniformly. Pass through suitable sieve and preserve in a well-closed container.

- **Storage:** Store in a well-closed container and protect from atmospheric moisture.

VIVA VOCE QUESTIONS

Q.1   What is the use of liquorice?

____

Q.2   What is the use of senna and fennel?

____

Q.3   Define laxative.

____

❖ ❖ ❖

Formulation Table:

Ingredients	Quantity required for 200 g	Quantity required for _____ g
Sodium chloride	50 g	_____ g
Potassium chloride	70 g	_____ g
Sodium bicarbonate	70 g	_____ g
Dextrose	10 g	_____ g

Calculations:

Sodium chloride required to prepare 200 g of powder = 50 g

So, for preparation of _____ g powder, Senna leaf powder required = $\dfrac{50}{200} \times$ —— = —— g

Potassium chloride required to prepare 200 g of powder = 70 g

So, for preparation of _____ g powder, Potassium chloride required = $\dfrac{70}{200} \times$ — = — g

Sodium bicarbonate quantity same as Potassium chloride = _____ g

Dextrose required to prepare 200 g of powder = 10 g

So, for preparation of _____ g powder, Dextrose required = $\dfrac{10}{200} \times$ —— = —— g

Label of Preparation:

ELECTROLYTE POWDER			
Each 200 g contains			
Sodium chloride : 50 g			
Potassium chloride : 70 g			
Sodium bicarbonate : 70 g			
Dextrose : 10 g			
Patient name:		**Age:**	
Sex:		**Weight:**	
Dose: As directed by the physician.			
Mfg. date:		**Exp. Date:**	
Batch no.:		**Price:**	
Prepared by:			

Date : _____________   Marks : _________/10

EXPERIMENT NO. 18

- **Aim:** To prepare _________ g electrolyte powder.

- **Theory:** Pharmaceutical powders are mixture of finely divided drugs or chemicals in dry forms. They are intended for internal or external use for many diseases. Pharmaceutical powders may be classified on the basis of dispensing of powders. These are bulk powder for external use, bulk powder for internal use, divided powder for internal use, effervescent powder or granules.

  Uses: Used for electrolyte balance and dehydration.

  Dose: As per need and response of patient.

- **Procedure:** Mix weighed amount of substances in ascending order of their weight. Wrap individual powder quantity in aluminium foil with inner wax lined paper.

- **Storage:** Store in a well-closed container and protect from atmospheric moisture.

VIVA VOCE QUESTIONS

Q.1   What is electrolyte?

____

Q.2   What are the elements which are most essential for body?

____

Q.3   How to prepare electrolyte powder?

____

❖ ❖ ❖

Formulation Table:

Ingredients	Quantity required for 100 ml	Quantity required for _____ ml
Chloroform	0.25 ml	_______ ml
Purified water sufficient to produce	100.0 ml	_______ ml

Calculations:

Chloroform required to prepare 100 ml of chloroform water = 0.25 ml

So, for preparation of _____ ml chloroform water, Chloroform required

$$= \frac{0.25}{100} \times \underline{\quad\quad} = \underline{\quad\quad} \text{ ml}$$

Label of Preparation:

CHLOROFORM WATER			
Each 100 ml contains			
Chloroform : 0.25 ml			
Purified Water : 100.0 ml			
Patient name:		**Age:**	
Sex:		**Weight:**	
Dose: As directed by the physician.			
Mfg. date:		**Exp. Date:**	
Batch no.:		**Price:**	
Prepared by:			

Date : ___________   Marks : ________/10

EXPERIMENT NO. 19

- **Aim:** To prepare _________ ml chloroform water.

- **Theory:** Aromatic waters are clear, saturated aqueous solutions of volatile oils or contain other aromatic or volatile substances. These are also known as medicated waters. Taste and odours of aromatic waters are similar to the drug or volatile substance which may incorporate in them. There are two official methods used to prepare aromatic waters : (a) Solution method and (b) Distillation method.

  Chloroform is a clear, odourless and a mobile liquid with ether odour and has burning sweet taste. Care should be taken in handling chloroform because in presence of flame or light, it produces harmful gases like hydrogen chloride and phosgene gases. The small amount of ethanol in chloroform retards the formation of carbonyl chloride. It is rarely used as inhalation anaesthetic due to its serious side effect on heart and liver. Internally in small dose it is used as carminative and externally it is used as irritant. In the preparation of chloroform water, vigorous shaking is necessary to subdivide the chloroform in small globules to enhance the solubility. In this preparation distributive agent is not required, as the product is half saturated with chloroform.

  Category: Pharmaceutical aid.

  Dose: 15 to 30 ml.

  Uses: Pharmaceutical aid, preservative, vehicle and general anaesthetic.

- **Procedure:** Measure the required amount of chloroform and dissolve it in purified water by shaking. Chloroform is completely dissolved in water. Transfer it in clean amber coloured container and close it tightly.

- **Storage:** Store in a well-closed container and protect from light.

VIVA VOCE QUESTIONS

Q.1   What is the use of chloroform water?

____

Q.2   Why chloroform is not used as an anaesthetic agent?

____

Q.3   Which method is used to prepare chloroform water?

____

❖ ❖ ❖

Formulation Table:

Ingredients	Quantity required for 100 ml	Quantity required for ______ ml
Camphor	0.10 g	______ g
Ethanol (90%)	0.20 ml	______ ml
Purified water sufficient to produce	100.0 ml	______ ml

Calculations:

Camphor required to prepare 100 ml of camphor water = 0.10 g

So, for preparation of ___ ml camphor water, Camphor required = $\dfrac{0.10}{100}$ × ____ = ____ g

Ethanol required to prepare 100 ml of camphor water = 0.20 ml

So, for preparation of ___ ml camphor water, Ethanol required = $\dfrac{0.20}{100}$ × ____ = ____ ml

Label of Preparation:

CAMPHOR WATER		
Each 100 ml contains Camphor : 0.10 g Ethanol : 0.20 ml Purified water : 100.0 ml		
Patient Name:	**Age:**	
Sex:	**Weight:**	
Dose: As directed by the physician.		
Mfg. Date:	**Exp. Date:**	
Batch No.:	**Price:**	
Prepared by:		

Date :____________   Marks : ________/10

EXPERIMENT NO. 20

- **Aim:** To prepare ________ ml camphor water.

- **Theory:** Aromatic waters are clear, saturated aqueous solutions of volatile oils or contain other aromatic or volatile substances. These are also known as medicated waters. Taste and odours of aromatic waters are similar to the drug or volatile substance which may incorporate in them. There are two official methods used to prepare aromatic waters : (a) Solution method and (b) Distillation method.

- Camphor is a ketone, obtained from *Cinnamomum camphora*. It is colourless or white crystals, granules or crystalline masses. It is highly volatile in nature at room temperature and readily burns with a bright smoky flame. It is soluble in 800 parts of water and in 1 part of ethanol. In the preparation of aromatic water, ethanol acts as distributing agent. Water cannot be added in alcoholic solution of camphor because if whole camphor is precipitated, then it becomes difficult to re-dissolve it by shaking the solution.

  Category: Pharmaceutical aid.

  Dose: 15 to 30 ml.

  Uses: Pharmaceutical aid, vehicle and is used as carminative and to relieve gripping pain.

- **Procedure:** Dissolve measured amount of camphor in ethanol. Add alcoholic solution dropwise in purified water with shaking. Afterwards shake occasionally until all the camphor is dissolved. If necessary, filter the solution and store in a closed container.

- **Storage:** Store in a well-closed container.

VIVA VOCE QUESTIONS

Q.1   What is camphor? Write its pharmaceutical applications.

____

Q.2   How camphor water is prepared?

____

Q.3   What is the use of ethanol in water for preparation of camphor water?

____

❖❖❖

Formulation Table:

Ingredients	Quantity required for 100 ml	Quantity required for _____ ml
Peppermint oil	2.0 ml	_____ ml
Ethanol (90%)	60.0 ml	_____ ml
Purified water sufficient to produce	100.0 ml	_____ ml

Calculations:

Peppermint oil required to prepare 100 ml of conc. peppermint water = 2.0 ml

So, for preparation of _____ ml conc. peppermint water, peppermint oil required

$$= \frac{2.0}{100} \times \text{\_\_\_\_\_} = \text{\_\_\_\_\_ ml}$$

Ethanol required to prepare 100 ml of conc. peppermint water = 60.0 ml

So, for preparation of _____ ml conc. peppermint water, ethanol required

$$= \frac{60.0}{100} \times \text{\_\_\_\_\_} = \text{\_\_\_\_\_ ml}$$

Label of Preparation:

CONCENTRATED PEPPERMINT WATER			
Each 100 ml contains			
Peppermint oil : 2.0 ml			
Ethanol : 60.0 ml			
Purified water : 100.0 ml			
Patient Name:		**Age:**	
Sex:		**Weight:**	
Dose: As directed by the physician.			
Mfg. Date:		**Exp. Date:**	
Batch No.:		**Price:**	
Prepared by:			

Date :___________   Marks : _________/10

EXPERIMENT NO. 21

- **Aim:** To prepare _________ ml concentrated peppermint water.
- **Theory:** Concentrated aromatic waters are alcoholic saturated solutions of volatile oils or other substances and are about 40 times stronger than the aromatic waters. Aromatic waters are prepared by diluting 1 part of concentrated aromatic water within 39 parts of water. In these preparations oil content is excess than that required to form a saturated solution. Purified talc is used as absorbent to remove excess amount of oil. The preparation is allowed to stand for a few hours to finely divided globules of oil to coalesce. Then it is shaked to enhance the absorption of the excessive or insoluble amount of oil. The aromatic part of the oil is soluble in the vehicle, while other non-aromatic part containing terpenes is insoluble in the vehicle. The undissolved non-aromatic part of the oil is separated along with the talc by filtration of water.

  Category: Pharmaceutical aid, flavouring agent.

  Dose: 0.25 – 1.0 ml.

  Uses: It is used as flavouring agent and carminative.

- **Procedure:** Dissolve measured amount of volatile oil in 90% ethanol. Add the sufficient purified water in successive small portion with vigorous shaking and make up the required volume. It is necessary to shake vigorously after each addition. Add 5.0 g of sterilized purified talc and shake it. Allow to stand for a few minutes and shake occasionally. Remove talc by filtration and store in a well-closed container.

- **Storage:** Store in a well-closed container.

VIVA VOCE QUESTIONS

Q.1   What is a peppermint? Give application of talc in peppermint water.

____

Q.2   How to prepare peppermint water?

____

Q.3   Give pharmaceutical application of aromatic water.

____

Q. 4   What is the use of ethanol in water in peppermint water?

____

❖ ❖ ❖

Formulation Table:

Ingredients	Quantity required for 100 ml	Quantity required for _____ ml
Benzaldehyde	1.0 ml	_______ ml
Ethanol (90%)	80.0 ml	_______ ml
Purified water, upto	100.0 ml	_______ ml

Calculations:

Benzaldehyde required to prepare 100 ml of spirit = 1.0 ml

So, for preparation of _____ ml spirit, Benzaldehyde required = $\dfrac{1.0}{100}$ × ——— = ——— ml

Ethanol required to prepare 100 ml of spirit = 80.0 ml

So, for preparation of _____ ml spirit, Ethanol required = $\dfrac{80.0}{100}$ × ——— = ——— ml

Label of Preparation:

BENZALDEHYDE SPIRIT			
Each 100 ml contains			
Benzaldehyde : 1.0 ml			
Ethanol (90%) : 80.0 ml			
Purified water, upto : 100.0 ml			
Patient Name:		**Age:**	
Sex:		**Weight:**	
Dose: As directed by the physician.			
Mfg. Date:		**Exp. Date:**	
Batch No.:		**Price:**	
Prepared by:			

Date :___________   Marks : ________/10

EXPERIMENT NO. 22

- **Aim:** To prepare _________ ml benzaldehyde spirit.

- **Theory:** Spirits are alcoholic or hydroalcoholic solutions of volatile substances and contain 50% to 90% of alcohol. The high alcoholic content maintains water-insoluble oils in solution. If water is added to the spirit, volatile oil starts to separate. Some spirits are used as a flavouring agents. Spirits are prepared by dissolving or distillation method.

  Benzaldehyde is a colourless, strongly refractive liquid and having an odour resembling that of bitter almond oil and a burning aromatic taste. It is also known as artificial essential almond oil. It is used in place of bitter almond oil for flavouring purposes. It is much safer than almond oil as it contains no hydrocynic acid. It is also used in perfumery and in manufacturing of dyestuff.

  Category: Flavouring agent.

  Uses: It is used as flavouring agent and perfuming agent.

- **Procedure:** Dissolve measured amount of benzaldehyde in ethanol (90%). Add sufficient purified water to make up the volume and mix properly by shaking.

- **Storage:** Benzaldehyde spirit should be kept in a well-filled container and protected from light.

VIVA VOCE QUESTIONS

Q.1   What is spirit?

____

Q.2   Why benzaldehyde spirit is needed?

____

Q.3   How spirits are prepared?

____

Q. 4.   Why do you prefer benzaldehyde than almond oil?

____

❖ ❖ ❖

Formulation Table:

Ingredients	Quantity required for 100 ml	Quantity required for _____ ml
Peppermint oil	10.0 ml	_______ ml
Ethanol (90%), upto	100.0 ml	_______ ml

Calculations:

Peppermint oil required to prepare 100 ml of spirit = 10.0 ml

So, for preparation of _____ ml spirit, Peppermint oil required = $\dfrac{10.0}{100}$ × ——— = ——— ml

Label of Preparation:

PEPPERMINT SPIRIT			
Each 100 ml contains			
Peppermint oil : 10.0 ml			
Ethanol (90%), upto : 100.0 ml			
Patient Name:		**Age:**	
Sex:		**Weight:**	
Dose: As directed by the physician.			
Mfg. Date:		**Exp. Date:**	
Batch No.:		**Price:**	
Prepared by:			

Date : _____________   Marks : _________/10

EXPERIMENT NO. 23

- **Aim:** To prepare ________ ml peppermint spirit.

- **Theory:** Spirits are alcoholic or hydroalcoholic solutions of volatile substances and contain 50% to 90% of alcohol. The high alcoholic content maintains water-insoluble oils in solution. If water is added to the spirit, volatile oil starts to separate. Some spirits are used as flavouring agents. Spirits are prepared by dissolving or distillation method.

  Peppermint oil is obtained by distillation from the fresh over-ground parts of the flowering plants of *Menthapiperita* Linn. It is a colourless or pale yellow liquid having a strong penetrating odour of peppermint and pungent taste, followed by a sensation of cold when air is drawn into the mouth. The odour of fresh peppermint is due to the presence of about 2.0% of a volatile oil, much of which is lost due to drying of leaves in air.

  Category: Flavouring agent and Carminative.

  Uses: It is used as flavouring agent, carminative, antiseptic and local anaesthetic.

  Dose: Usually 1 ml three times a day.

- **Procedure:** Take measured quantity of peppermint oil and mix with ethanol. If the solution is not clear, shake with purified talc (5%) and filter it. Add sufficient amount of ethanol to make up the volume.

- **Storage:** Store in a well-closed container and in a cool place.

VIVA VOCE QUESTIONS

Q.1   What is the source of peppermint oil?

____

Q.2   How peppermint spirit is prepared?

____

Q.3   What is the role of talc in the preparation of spirit?

____

Q. 4.   Give storage condition of spirit.

____

❖ ❖ ❖

Formulation Table:

Ingredients	Quantity required for 100 ml
Belladona herb in moderate coarse powder	100.0 g
Ethanol (70%), upto	100.0 ml

Label of Preparation:

BELLADONA TINCTURE			
Each 100 ml contains			
Belladona herb : 100 g			
Ethanol (90%), upto : 100.0 ml			
Patient Name:		**Age:**	
Sex:		**Weight:**	
Dose: As directed by the physician.			
Mfg. Date:		**Exp. Date:**	
Batch No.:		**Price:**	
Prepared by:			

Date :___________   Marks : ________/10

EXPERIMENT NO. 24

- **Aim:** To prepare 100 ml belladona tincture.

- **Theory:** Tincture is defined as alcoholic or hydroalcoholic solution prepared from vegetable materials or from chemical substances. Tinctures are generally prepared by two methods:

  1. **Percolation:** This method is most frequently used to extract the active ingredients in the preparation of tinctures and fluid extracts. It contains a narrow cone-shaped vessel open at both ends, known as percolator. The solid substances are moistened with a suitable amount of specified menstrum and are allowed to stand for about three to four hours. The mass with menstrum is saturated in percolator and allowed to macerate in closed percolator for 24 hours. The outlet of the percolator is then opened and the liquid is allowed to drip slowly. If necessary, additional menstrum is added until the volume of the percolate collected is about three quarters of the liquid. The mixture of various portions of percolate is clarified by filtration.

  2. **Maceration:** In this process, the solid substances are placed in a stopper container with the whole of the solvent and are allowed to stand for a period of at least three days. Then the solvent is strained and marc is pressed and combined with extract liquid.

  Uses: It is used as a parasympatholytic.

- **Procedure:** Prepare the tincture by percolation. Determine the proportion of alkaloids in the tincture by assay. It contains in 2.0 ml, 0.6 mg of alkaloid of belladonna. Add sufficient ethanol to produce a sufficient strength of belladonna. Keep aside twenty four hours and then filter.

  Dose: 0.6 to 2.0 ml.

- **Storage:** Store in an air tight container and protect from light.

VIVA VOCE QUESTIONS

Q.1   What is tincture?

____

Q.2   How belladonna tincture is prepared?

____

Q.3   What is percolation?

____

❖ ❖ ❖

Formulation Table:

Ingredients	Quantity required for 100 ml
Cardamom oil	0.3 ml
Carraway oil	1.0 ml
Cinnamon oil	1.0 ml
Clove oil	1.0 ml
Strong ginger tincture	6.0 ml
Ethanol (90%), upto	100.0 ml

Label of Preparation:

CARDMAMOM TINCTURE			
Each 100 ml contains			
Cardamom oil	: 0.3 ml		
Carraway oil	: 1.0 ml		
Cinnamon oil	: 1.0 ml		
Clove oil	: 1.0 ml		
Strong ginger tincture	: 6.0 ml		
Ethanol (90%), upto	: 100.0 ml		
Patient Name:		**Age:**	
Sex:		**Weight:**	
Dose: As directed by the physician.			
Mfg. Date:		**Exp. Date:**	
Batch No.:		**Price:**	
Prepared by:			

Date :___________   Marks : _______/10

EXPERIMENT NO. 25

- **Aim:** To prepare 100 ml aromatic cardamom tincture.
- **Theory:** Tincture is defined as alcoholic or hydroalcoholic solution prepared from vegetable materials or from chemical substances. Tinctures are generally prepared by two methods :

  1. **Percolation:** This method is most frequently used to extract the active ingredients in the preparation of tinctures and fluid extracts. It contains a narrow cone-shaped vessel open at both ends known as percolator. The solid substances are moistened with a suitable amount of specified menstrum and are allowed to stand for about three to four hours. The mass with menstrum is saturated in percolator and allowed to macerate in closed percolator for 24 hours. The outlet of the percolator is then opened and the liquid is allowed to drip slowly. If necessary, additional menstrum is added until the volume of the percolate collected is about three quarters of the liquid. The mixture of various portions of percolate is clarified by filtration.

  2. **Maceration:** In this process, the solid substances are placed in a stopper container with the whole of the solvent and are allowed to stand for a period of at least three days. Then the solvent is strained and marc is pressed and combined with extract liquid.

  Uses: It is used as a carminative.

- **Procedure:** Moisten the mixed powders with a sufficient quantity of alcohol and prepare about 900 ml of tincture by percolation. Add glycerin and mix. Add solution of amaranth. Add sufficient ethanol to produce 100 ml tincture. Filter the tincture and preserve in a suitable container.

- **Dose:** 2 to 4 ml.

- **Storage:** Preserve in a well-closed container.

VIVA VOCE QUESTIONS

Q.1   What are differences between tinctures and extracts?

____

Q.2   How to prepare tinctures?

____

Q.3   What are the pharmaceutical uses of tincture?

____

❖❖❖

Formulation Table:

Ingredients	Quantity required for 100 ml
Fresh orange peel in the slices	25.0 g
Ethanol (90%) , upto	100.0 ml

Label of Preparation:

ORANGE TINCTURE			
Each 100 ml contains			
Fresh orange peel　　　: 25.0 g			
Ethanol (90%), upto　　: 100.0 ml			
Patient Name:		**Age:**	
Sex:		**Weight:**	
Dose: As directed by the physician.			
Mfg. Date:		**Exp. Date:**	
Batch No.:		**Price:**	
Prepared by:			

Date :___________   Marks : _________/10

EXPERIMENT NO. 26

- **Aim:** To prepare 100 ml orange tincture.

- **Theory:** Tincture is defined as alcoholic or hydroalcoholic solution prepared from vegetable materials or from chemical substances. Tinctures are generally prepared by two methods :

  1. **Percolation:** This method is most frequently used to extract the active ingredients in the preparation of tinctures and fluid extracts. It contains a narrow cone-shaped vessel open at both ends, known as percolator. The solid substances are moistened with a suitable amount of specified menstrum and are allowed to stand for about three to four hours. The mass with menstrum is saturated in percolator and allowed to macerate in closed percolator for 24 hours. The outlet of the percolator is then opened and the liquid is allowed to drip slowly. If necessary, additional menstrum is added until the volume of the percolate collected is about three quarters of the liquid. The mixture of various portions of percolate is clarified by filtration.

  2. **Maceration:** In this process, the solid substances are placed in a stopper container with the whole of the solvent and are allowed to stand for a period of at least three days. Then the solvent is strained and marc is pressed and combined with extract liquid.

  Uses: It is used as a flavouring agent.

- **Procedure:** Prepare the tincture by percolation process. Add sufficient amount of ethanol to produce required volume of tincture.

  Dose: 2 to 4 ml.

- **Storage:** Preserve in a well-closed container.

VIVA VOCE QUESTIONS

Q.1   How to preserve the tinctures?

____

Q.2   How to prepare orange tincture?

____

Q.3   What are the pharmaceutical uses of tincture?

____

❖❖❖

Formulation Table:

Ingredients	Quantity required for 100 ml
Cardamom seed in powder form	1.4 g
Caraway in powder form	1.4 g
Cinnamon in powder form	2.8 g
Amaranth	0.50 g
Glycerin	5.0 ml
Ethanol (90%), upto	100.0 ml

Label of Preparation:

CARDAMOM EXTRACT		
Each 100 ml contains		
Cardamom Seed in powder form : 1.4 g		
Caraway in powder form : 1.4 g		
Cinnamon in powder form : 2.8 g		
Amaranth : 0.50 g		
Glycerin : 5.0 ml		
Ethanol (90%), upto : 100.0 ml		
Patient Name:	**Age:**	
Sex:	**Weight:**	
Dose: As directed by the physician.		
Mfg. Date:	**Exp. Date:**	
Batch No.:	**Price:**	
Prepared by:		

Date :___________   Marks : _________/10

EXPERIMENT NO. 27

- **Aim:** To prepare 100 ml compound cardamom extract.

- **Theory:** Extraction, as the term is used pharmaceutically, involves the separation of medicinally active portions of plant or animal tissues from the inactive or inert components by using selective solvents in standard extraction procedures. The products so obtained from plants are relatively impure liquids, semisolids or powders intended only for oral or external use. These include classes of preparations known as decoctions, infusions, fluid extracts, tinctures, pilular (semisolid) extracts and powdered extracts. Such preparations popularly have been called galenicals, named after Galen, the second century Greek physician. The purposes of standardized extraction procedures for crude drugs are to attain the therapeutically desired portion and to eliminate the inert material by treatment with a selective solvent known as menstrum. The extract thus obtained may be ready for use as a medicinal agent in the form of tinctures and fluid extracts, it may be further processed to be incorporated in any dosage form such as tablets or capsules, or it may be fractionated to isolate individual chemical entities such as ajmalicine, hyoscine and vincristine, which are modern drugs. Thus, standardization of extraction procedures contributes significantly to the final quality of the herbal drug.

  Uses: It is used as a carminative.

- **Procedure:** Moisten the mixed powders with a sufficient quantity of alcohol and prepare about 100 ml of extract by percolation method. Add glycerin and mix. Add solution of amaranth. Add sufficient ethanol to produce required tincture. Filter the tincture and preserve in a suitable container.

  Dose: 2 to 4 ml

- **Storage:** Preserve in a well-closed container.

VIVA VOCE QUESTIONS

Q.1   What are the differences between tinctures and extracts?

____

Q.2   How to prepare extracts?

____

Q.3   What are the pharmaceutical uses of extracts?

____

❖❖❖

Formulation Table:

Ingredients	Quantity required for 100 ml
Fresh orange peel in the slices	25.0 g
Ethanol (90%) , upto	100.0 ml

Label of Preparation:

ORANGE EXTRACT			
Each 100 ml contains			
Fresh orange peel : 25.0 g			
Ethanol (90%), upto : 100.0 ml			
Patient Name:		**Age:**	
Sex:		**Weight:**	
Dose: As directed by the physician.			
Mfg. Date:		**Exp. Date:**	
Batch No.:		**Price:**	
Prepared by:			

Date :_____________   Marks : _________/10

EXPERIMENT NO. 28

- **Aim:** To prepare 100 ml orange extract.

- **Theory:** Extraction, as the term is used pharmaceutically, involves the separation of medicinally active portions of plant or animal tissues from the inactive or inert components by using selective solvents in standard extraction procedures. The products so obtained from plants are relatively impure liquids, semisolids or powders intended only for oral or external use. These include classes of preparations known as decoctions, infusions, fluid extracts, tinctures, pilular (semisolid) extracts and powdered extracts. Such preparations popularly have been called galenicals, named after Galen, the second century Greek physician. The purposes of standardized extraction procedures for crude drugs are to attain the therapeutically desired portion and to eliminate the inert material by treatment with a selective solvent known as menstrum. The extract thus obtained may be ready for use as a medicinal agent in the form of tinctures and fluid extracts, it may be further processed to be incorporated in any dosage form such as tablets or capsules, or it may be fractionated to isolate individual chemical entities such as ajmalicine, hyoscine and vincristine, which are modern drugs. Thus, standardization of extraction procedures contributes significantly to the final quality of the herbal drug.

  Uses: It is used as a flavouring agent.

- **Procedure:** Prepare the extract by percolation process. Add sufficient amount of ethanol to produce required extract.

  Dose: 2 to 4 ml.

- **Storage:** Preserve in a well-closed container.

VIVA VOCE QUESTIONS

Q.1   How to preserve the extracts?

____

Q.2   How to prepare orange extract?

____

Q.3   What are the pharmaceutical uses of extracts?

____

❖ ❖ ❖

Formulation Table:

Ingredients	Quantity required for 100 ml	Quantity required for _____ ml
Cresol	50.0 ml	_______ ml
Vegetable oil	18.0 g	_______ g
Potassium hydroxide	4.20 g	_______ g
Purified water sufficient to produce	100.0 ml	_______ ml

Calculations:

Cresol required to prepare 100 ml of solution = 50.0 ml

So, for preparation of _____ ml solution, cresol required = $\dfrac{50.0}{100} \times$ —— = —— ml

Vegetable oil required to prepare 100 ml of solution = 18.0 g

So, for preparation of _____ ml solution, vegetable oil required = $\dfrac{18.0}{100} \times$ —— = —— g

Potassium hydroxide required to prepare 100 ml of solution = 4.20 g

So, for preparation of _____ ml solution, Potassium hydroxide required = $\dfrac{4.20}{100} \times$ —— = —— g

Label of Preparation:

CRESOL SOAP SOLUTION			
Each 100 ml contains			
Cresol	: 50.0 ml		
Vegetable oil	: 18.0 g		
Potassium hydroxide	: 4.20 g		
Purified water, upto	: 100.0 ml		
Patient Name:		**Age:**	
Sex:		**Weight:**	
Dose: As directed by the physician.			
Mfg. Date:		**Exp. Date:**	
Batch No.:		**Price:**	
Prepared by:			

Date :___________   Marks : ________/10

EXPERIMENT NO. 29

- **Aim:** To prepare ________ ml cresol with soap solution.

- **Theory:** A solution is a homogeneous one phase system consisting of two or more components. It contains two phases i.e. solvent and solute. The solvent is the phase in which the dispersion occurs and solute is that component which is dispersed as small ions or molecules in the solvents. The advantages of solutions are: (i) Easy to swallow. (ii) Suitable for paediatric preparations. (iii) Drug in solution form is readily available for absorption.

  Cresol is a mixture of ortho, meta and para-cresol. It acts as a disinfectant. The solubility of cresol in water is only about 3%; whereas the quantity of cresol present in this preparation is 50%. For dissolving this high proportion of cresol, solubilising agent is required. Fatty acids containing vegetable oil react with hydroxide and form soap. This soap also acts as solubilising agent. The reaction between vegetable oil and potassium hydroxide can be enhanced by adding small amount of ethyl alcohol. Cresol is a phenolic compound and caustic in nature, therefore, it should be handled carefully.

  Category: Disinfectant.

- **Procedure:** Dissolve potassium hydroxide in 25 ml of purified water. Add vegetable oil and heat on a water-bath. Mix thoroughly. Continue heating until a small portion dissolves in water without separation of oily drops. Add cresol and mix thoroughly. Add sufficient purified water to produce the required volume.

- **Storage:** Preserve in a narrow-mouthed bottle.

VIVA VOCE QUESTIONS

Q.1   What are solutions?

____

Q.2   How cresol with soap solution is prepared?

____

Q.3   What are disinfectants?

____

Q. 4.   What is lysol?

____

❖❖❖

Formulation Table:

Ingredients	Quantity required for 100 ml	Quantity required for _____ ml
Iodine	10.0 g	_____ g
Potassium iodide	6.0 g	_____ g
Purified water	10.0 ml	_____ ml
Ethanol, upto	100.0 ml	_____ ml

Calculations:

Iodine required to prepare 100 ml of solution = 10.0 g

So, for preparation of _____ ml solution, Iodine required = $\dfrac{10.0}{100} \times$ —— = —— g

Potassium iodide required to prepare 100 ml of solution = 6.0 g

So, for preparation of _____ ml solution, Potassium iodide required = $\dfrac{6.0}{100} \times$ —— = —— g

Purified water required to prepare 100 ml of solution = 10.0 ml

So, for preparation of _____ ml solution, water required = $\dfrac{10.0}{100} \times$ —— = —— ml

Label of Preparation:

STRONG IODINE SOLUTION			
Each 100 ml contains			
Iodine : 10.0 g			
Potassium iodide : 6.0 g			
Purified water : 10.0 ml			
Ethanol, upto : 100.0 ml			
Patient Name:		**Age:**	
Sex:		**Weight:**	
Dose: As directed by the physician.			
Mfg. Date:		**Exp. Date:**	
Batch No.:		**Price:**	
Prepared by:			

Date :___________   Marks : _________/10

EXPERIMENT NO. 30

- **Aim:** To prepare _________ ml strong iodine solution.

- **Theory:** A solution is a homogeneous one phase system consisting of two or more components. It contains two phases i.e. solvent and solute. The solvent is the phase in which the dispersion occurs and solute is that component which is dispersed as small ions or molecules in the solvents. The advantages of solutions are: (i) Easy to swallow. (ii) Suitable for paediatric preparations. (iii) Drug in solution form is readily available for absorption.

  In 1829, a French professor by the name of J.G.A. Lugol mixed water, potassium iodide and iodine to make what is called Lugol's iodine. When testing for starch, if any is present, it will turn a dark blue to black colour. This is caused by polysaccharides reacting with iodine. Simple sugars cannot be detected using Lugol's iodine. Lugol's iodine solution is often used as an antiseptic and disinfectant, for emergency disinfection of drinking water, and as a reagent for starch detection in routine laboratory and medical tests. These uses are possible since the solution is a source of effectively free elemental iodine, which is readily generated from the equilibrium between elemental iodine molecules and triiodide ion in the solution.

  Category: Antiseptic.

- **Procedure:** Mix potassium iodide and iodine in glass pestle motor. Dissolve potassium iodide and iodine mixture in a purified water. Add sufficient ethanol to produce required volume.

- **Storage:** Preserve strong iodine solution in a well-closed container. The material of the container should be resistant to iodine.

VIVA VOCE QUESTIONS

Q.1   What are the uses of iodine?

____

Q.2   What is the use of potassium iodide in this solution?

____

Q.3   How strong iodine solution is prepared?

____

Q. 4   What are the differences between antiseptic and disinfectant?

____

❖❖❖

Formulation Table:

Ingredients	Quantity required for 100 ml	Quantity required for _____ ml
Lead acetate	25.0 g	_____ g
Lead monoxide in powder	17.5 g	_____ g
Purified water, upto	100 ml	_____ ml

Calculations:

Lead acetate required to prepare 100 ml of solution = 25.0 g

So, for preparation of _____ ml solution, Lead acetate required = $\dfrac{25.0}{100}$ × —— = —— g

Lead monoxide required to prepare 100 ml of solution = 17.5 g

So, for preparation of _____ ml solution, Lead monoxide required = $\dfrac{17.5}{100}$ × —— = —— g

Purified water required to prepare 100 ml of solution = 100 ml

So, for preparation of _____ ml solution, water required = $\dfrac{100}{100}$ × —— = —— ml

Label of Preparation:

STRONG LEAD ACETATE SOLUTION			
Each 100 ml contains			
Lead acetate : 25. 0 g			
Lead monoxide : 17.5 g			
Purified water, upto : 100.0 ml			
Patient Name:		**Age:**	
Sex:		**Weight:**	
Dose: As directed by the physician.			
Mfg. Date:		**Exp. Date:**	
Batch No.:		**Price:**	
Prepared by:			

Date :___________   Marks : _________/10

EXPERIMENT NO. 31

- **Aim:** To prepare _______ ml strong lead acetate solution.

- **Theory:** A solution is a homogeneous one phase system consisting of two or more components. It contains two phases i.e. solvent and solute. The solvent is the phase in which the dispersion occurs and solute is that component which is dispersed as small ions or molecules in the solvents.

  Lead monoxide and lead acetate react together and form a number of basic lead acetates. The basic lead acetate is formed by the following reaction :

$$(CH_3COO)_2Pb + PbO \longrightarrow (CH_3COO)_2Pb . Pb(OH)_2$$

  This basic acetate of lead is soluble in water. Highly alkaline solution of acetate of lead $(CH_3COO)_2Pb.Pb(OH)_2$ is poorly soluble. Filtration should be conducted as quickly as possible and preferably performed into a bottle in such a manner that the filtrate should not expose to carbon dioxide any longer than required, because carbon dioxide of atmosphere precipitates the basic lead acetate and converts insoluble basic lead carbonate. For the same reason, the preparation is stored in small bottles which are well- filled and well-closed.

  Category: Antiseptic.

  Uses: Soothing astringent.

- **Procedure:** Dissolve lead acetate in small quantity of purified water. Add lead monoxide. Set aside for forty-eight hours. Shake occasionally and pass the solution through the filter. Add sufficient purified water to produce required volume.

- **Storage:** Preserve in a well-filled and well-closed container.

VIVA VOCE QUESTIONS

Q.1   What is the chemical reaction of lead acetate?

____

Q.2   What are the uses of lead acetate solution?

____

Q.3   How lead acetate solution is prepared?

____

Q. 4   What are the differences between solution and mixture?

____

❖ ❖ ❖

Formulation Table:

Ingredients	Quantity required for 100 ml	Quantity required for _____ ml
Sodium chloride	8.6 g	______ g
Potasium chloride	0.3 g	______ g
Calcium chloride hydrated	0.33 g	______ g
Purified water, upto	100.0 ml	______ ml

Calculations:

Sodium chloride required to prepare 100 ml of solution = 8.6 g

So, for preparation of _____ ml solution, Sodium chloride required $= \dfrac{8.6}{100} \times — = — $ g

Potassium chloride required to prepare 100 ml of solution = 0.3 g

So, for preparation of _____ ml solution, potassium chloride required $= \dfrac{0.3}{100} \times — = — $ g

Calcium chloride required to prepare 100 ml of solution = 0.33 g

So, for preparation of _____ ml solution, Calcium chloride required $= \dfrac{0.33}{100} \times — = — $ g

Label of Preparation:

COMPOUND SODIUM CHLORIDE SOLUTION			
Each 100 ml contains			
Sodium chloride : 8.6 g			
Potasium chloride : 0.3 g			
Calcium chloride hydrated : 0.33 g			
Purified water, upto : 100.0 ml			
Patient Name:		**Age:**	
Sex:		**Weight:**	
Dose: As directed by the physician.			
Mfg. Date:		**Exp. Date:**	
Batch No.:		**Price:**	
Prepared by:			

Date :___________   Marks : _________/10

EXPERIMENT NO. 32

- **Aim:** To prepare _________ ml compound sodium chloride solution.

- **Theory:** A solution is a homogeneous one phase system consisting of two or more components. It contains two phases i.e. solvent and solute. The solvent is the phase in which the dispersion occurs and solute is that component which is dispersed as small ions or molecules in the solvents.

  Compound sodium chloride is an isotonic solution of sodium chloride, potassium chloride and calcium chloride. It is used as fluid and electrolyte replenisher to irrigate the tissue during experiments on animals. Ringer's injection has the same composition except water for injection in place of purified water, when it is used during cardio pulmonary bypass heart surgery.

  Category: Fluid replenisher.

  Uses: Fluid and electrolyte replenisher.

- **Procedure:** Dissolve sodium chloride, potassium chloride and calcium chloride hydrated in a sufficient quantity of recently boiled purified water. Add purified water to make up the volume.

- **Storage:** Preserve in a well-closed container. Always freshly prepared solution is used.

VIVA VOCE QUESTIONS

Q.1   What is ringer's solution?

____

Q.2   How ringer's solution is prepared?

____

Q.3   Which three salts are used in this solution?

____

Q. 4.   Write the storage of ringer's solution.

____

❖❖❖

Formulation Table:

Ingredients	Quantity required for 100 ml	Quantity required for _____ ml
Potassium permanganate	25.0 g	_____ g
Purified water (qs)	100.0 ml	_____ ml

Calculations:

Potassium permanganate required to prepare 100 ml of gargles = 25.0 g

So, for preparation of _____ g gargles, Potassium permanganate required

$$= \frac{25}{100} \times \underline{\quad} = \underline{\quad} g$$

Label of Preparation:

POTASSIUM PERMANGANATE GARGLES			
Each 100 ml contains			
Potassium permanganate : 25.0 g			
Purified water (qs) : 100.0 ml			
Patient Name:		**Age:**	
Sex:		**Weight:**	
Dose: As directed by the physician.			
Mfg. Date:		**Exp. Date:**	
Batch No.:		**Price:**	
Prepared by:			

Date : ___________   Marks : _________/10

EXPERIMENT NO. 33

- **Aim:** To prepare _________ ml potassium permanganate gargles.
- **Theory:** Gargles are aqueous solutions used for treating the pharynx and nasopharynx by forcing air from lungs through the gargles that is held in the throat. Gargles are generally dispensed in concentrated form. They must be diluted with water prior to its use. Gargles are pleasantly flavoured and medicated than mouthwashes. Many mouthwashes are used as gargles, either as such or diluted with purified warm water. Gargles contain following substances viz.
  - Antibiotics
  - Antiseptics
  - Anti-inflammatory
  - Anti-fungal
  - Analgesics
  - Astringents
  - Alkalizing agents
  - Deodorants
  - Local anaesthetics

  Uses: Astringent.
- **Procedure:** Grind weighed amount of potassium permanganate with water. Remove undissolved permanganate by filtration and add sufficient amount of purified water to produce required quantity.
- **Storage:** Store in a well-closed container.

VIVA VOCE QUESTIONS

Q.1   What are gargles?

____

Q.2   What is the role of gargles in the cosmetics?

____

Q.3   Write difference between mouthwashes and gargles.

____

Q. 4.   Gargles contain which type of substances?

____

❖❖❖

Formulation Table:

Ingredients	Quantity required for 100 ml	Quantity required for _____ ml
Sodium bicarbonate	1.0 g	_______ g
Sodium chloride	1.5 g	_______ g
Conc. peppermint emulsion	2.5 ml	_______ ml
DS chloroform water	50.0 ml	_______ ml
Purified water	100.0 ml	_______ ml

Calculations:

Sodium bicarbonate required to prepare 100 ml of mouthwashes = 1.0 g

So, for preparation of ___ ml mouthwash, Sodium bicarbonate required $= \dfrac{1.0}{100} \times \underline{\quad\quad} = \underline{\quad\quad}$ g

Sodium chloride required to prepare 100 ml of mouthwashes = 1.5 g

So, for preparation of ___ ml mouthwash, Sodium chloride required $= \dfrac{1.5}{100} \times \underline{\quad\quad} = \underline{\quad\quad}$ g

Peppermint emulsion required to prepare 100 ml of mouthwashes = 2.5 ml

So, for preparation of ___ ml mouthwash, peppermint emulsion required $= \dfrac{2.5}{100} \times \underline{\quad\quad} = \underline{\quad\quad}$ ml

Chloroform water required to prepare 100 ml of mouthwashes = 50.0 ml

So, for preparation of ___ ml mouthwash, chloroform water required $= \dfrac{50}{100} \times \underline{\quad\quad} = \underline{\quad\quad}$ ml

Label of Preparation:

SODIUM CHLORIDE MOUTHWASH			
Each 100 ml contains			
Sodium bicarbonate	: 1.0 g		
Sodium chloride	: 1.5 g		
Conc. peppermint emulsion	: 2.5 ml		
DS Chloroform water	: 50.0 ml		
Purified water	: 100.0 ml		
Patient Name:		**Age:**	
Sex:		**Weight:**	
Dose: As directed by the physician.			
Mfg. Date:		**Exp. Date:**	
Batch No.:		**Price:**	
Prepared by:			

Date :___________   Marks : ________/10

EXPERIMENT NO. 34

- **Aim:** To prepare ________ ml compound sodium chloride mouthwash.

- **Theory:** A mouthwash is an aqueous solution which is most often used for its deodorant, refreshing or antiseptic effect. It may contain alcohol, glycerin, synthetic sweeteners, surface active agents, flavouring agents and colouring agents. Mouthwashes generally contain following substances :

  - Antibacterial agents: Alkaline phenol, hydrogen peroxide, buffered sodium perborate, thymol glycerin.

  - Astringents: Zinc sulphate, zinc chloride etc.

  - Flavouring agents

  - Deodorants

  Uses: Antipruritic.

- **Procedure:** Dissolve sodium bicarbonate and sodium chloride in purified water. Add concentrated peppermint emulsion and mix. Add double strength chloroform water. Add sufficient purified water to produce required volume.

- **Storage:** Store in a well-closed container.

VIVA VOCE QUESTIONS

Q.1   What are mouthwashes?

____

Q.2   How to prepare mouthwashes?

____

Q.3   What is the use of mouthwashes?

____

Q. 4   Mouthwashes contain which type of substances?

____

❖ ❖ ❖

Formulation Table:

Ingredients	Quantity required for 100 ml	Quantity required for _____ ml
Cetylpyridinium chloride	0.10 g	_____ g
Citric Acid	0.10 g	_____ g
Sodium saccharin	0.04 g	_____ g
Peppermint oil	0.15 ml	_____ ml
Polyoxyethylene sorbiton monostearate	0.3 g	_____ g
Ethanol	10.0 ml	_____ ml
Sorbitol solution	20.0 ml	_____ ml
Purified water	100.0 ml	_____ ml

Calculations:

Cetylpyridinium chloride required to prepare 100 ml of mouthwashes = 0.1 g

So, for preparation of __ ml, Cetylpyridinium chloride required $= \dfrac{0.1}{100} \times \text{---} = \text{---} $ g

Citric acid required to prepare 100 ml of mouthwashes = 0.1 g

So, for preparation of _____ ml mouthwash, Citric acid required $= \dfrac{0.1}{100} \times \text{---} = \text{---} $ g

Sodium saccharin required to prepare 100 ml of mouthwashes = 0.04 g

So, for preparation of ___ ml mouthwash, Sodium saccharin required $= \dfrac{0.04}{100} \times \text{---} = \text{---} $ g

Sorbitol solution required to prepare 100 ml of mouthwashes = 20.0 ml

So, for preparation of __ ml mouthwash, Sorbitol solution required $= \dfrac{20}{100} \times \text{---} = \text{---} $ ml

Label of Preparation:

CETYLPYRIDINIUM CHLORIDE MOUTHWASH			
Each 100 ml contains			
Cetylpyridinium chloride	: 0.10 g		
Citric acid	: 0.10 g		
Sodium saccharin	: 0.04 g		
Peppermint oil	: 0.15 ml		
Polyoxyethylene sorbiton monostearate	: 0.3 g		
Ethanol	: 10.0 ml		
Sorbitol solution	: 20.0 ml		
Purified water	: 100.0 ml		
Patient Name:		**Age:**	
Sex:		**Weight:**	
Dose: As directed by the physician.			
Mfg. Date:		**Exp. Date:**	
Batch No.:		**Price:**	
Prepared by:			

Date :___________								Marks : ________/10

EXPERIMENT NO. 35

- **Aim:** To prepare ________ ml cetylpyridinium chloride mouthwash.
- **Theory:** A mouthwash is an aqueous solution which is most often used for its deodorant, refreshing or antiseptic effect. It may contain alcohol, glycerin, synthetic sweeteners, surface active agents, flavouring agents and colouring agents. Mouthwashes generally contain following substances.
  - Antibacterial agents: Alkaline phenol, hydrogen peroxide, buffered sodium perborate, thymol glycerin.
  - Astringents: Zinc sulphate, zinc chloride, etc.
  - Flavouring agents
  - Deodorants
  - Cetylpyridinium chloride is used as antimicrobial agent and also contributes to the solubilising power of the system. This preparation contains low concentration of surfactant because the sorbitol contributes the solubilisation efficacy of this mouthwash.

  Uses: Local anti-infective and antiseptic.
- **Procedure:** Dissolve cetylpyridinium chloride, citric acid and sodium saccharin in a sufficient amount of the water and add ethanol. Mix polyoxyethelene sorbiton monostearate and flavour oils. Add slowly hydroalcoholic solution with stirring. Add sorbitol and mix. Add sufficient amount of purified water to produce required quantity.
- **Storage:** Preserve in a well-closed container.

VIVA VOCE QUESTIONS

Q.1	What are mouthwashes?

____

Q.2	Why surfactants are used in mouthwashes?

____

Q.3	How mouthwash is prepared?

____

Q. 4.	What will happen if mouthwash is taken orally?

____

❖❖❖

Formulation Table:

Ingredients	Quantity required for 10 ml	Quantity required for _____ ml
Zinc sulphate	25.0 mg	______ mg
Phenyl mercuric nitrate	80.0 mg	______ mg
Purified water	10.0 ml	______ ml

Calculations:

Zinc sulphate required to prepare 10 ml of solution = 25.0 mg

So, for preparation of _____ ml solution, Zinc sulphate required $= \dfrac{25}{10} \times$ —— $=$ —— mg

Phenyl mercuric nitrate required to prepare 10 ml of solution = 80.0 mg

So, for preparation of ___ ml solution, Phenyl mercuric nitrate required $= \dfrac{80}{10} \times$ — $=$ — g

Label of Preparation:

<table>
<tr><td colspan="4" align="center">ZINC SULPHATE EYE DROP</td></tr>
<tr><td colspan="4">Each 10 ml contains</td></tr>
<tr><td colspan="4">Zinc sulphate   : 25 mg</td></tr>
<tr><td colspan="4">Phenyl mercuric nitrate   : 80.0 mg</td></tr>
<tr><td colspan="4">Purified water   : 10.0 ml</td></tr>
<tr><td>Patient Name:</td><td></td><td>Age:</td><td></td></tr>
<tr><td>Sex:</td><td></td><td>Weight:</td><td></td></tr>
<tr><td colspan="4">Dose: As directed by the physician.</td></tr>
<tr><td>Mfg. Date:</td><td></td><td>Exp. Date:</td><td></td></tr>
<tr><td>Batch No.:</td><td></td><td>Price:</td><td></td></tr>
<tr><td colspan="4">Prepared by:

</td></tr>
</table>

Date :___________   Marks : ________/10

EXPERIMENT NO. 36

- **Aim:** To prepare ________ ml zinc sulphate eye drops.

- **Theory:** Ophthalmic preparations are sterile products, essentially free from foreign particles, suitably formulated and packaged in suitable container for either topical application to the eyelids or instillation into cul-de-sac between eyeball and eyelid.

  Eye drops are sterile, aqueous or oily solutions or suspensions of one or more medicaments intended for installation into the eye sac for diagnostic or therapeutic purposes.

  Zinc sulphate eye drops are sterile solutions of zinc sulphate containing phenylmercuric acetate or phenylmercuric nitrate as an anti-microbial agent. Zinc sulphate is colourless, crystalline powder in nature. It is efflorescent in dry air.

  Uses: Astringent.

- **Procedure:** Dissolve weighed amount of zinc sulphate in purified water with aseptic precautions. Dissolve phenylmercuric nitrate in small amount of purified water. Add this solution and mix. If required, filter it aseptically.

  Dose: One or two drops

- **Storage:** Preserve in a well-closed dropper container.

VIVA VOCE QUESTIONS

Q.1   What are eye drops?

____

Q.2   What are pharmaceutical applications of zinc sulphate?

____

Q.3   What are astringents?

____

Q. 4.   How eye drops are sterilized?

____

❖❖❖

Formulation Table:

Ingredients	Quantity required for 100 g	Quantity required for _____ g
Wool fat	10.0 g	_____ g
Yellow soft paraffin	80.0 g	_____ g
Liquid paraffin (qs)	100.0 g	_____ g

Calculations:

Wool fat required to prepare 100 g of ointment = 10.0 g

So, for preparation of _____ g eye ointment, Wool fat required $= \dfrac{10}{100} \times$ ——— $=$ ——— g

Yellow soft paraffin required to prepare 100 g of ointment = 80.0 g

So, for preparation of _____ g eye ointment, Yellow soft paraffin required

$$= \dfrac{80}{100} \times \text{———} = \text{———} \ g$$

Label of Preparation:

SIMPLE EYE OINTMENT			
Each 100 g contains			
Wool fat	: 10.0 g		
Yellow soft paraffin	: 80.0 g		
Liquid paraffin (qs)	: 100.0 g		
Patient Name:		**Age:**	
Sex:		**Weight:**	
Dose: As directed by the physician.			
Mfg. Date:		**Exp. Date:**	
Batch No.:		**Price:**	
Prepared by:			

Date :____________   Marks : ________/10

EXPERIMENT NO. 37

- **Aim:** To prepare ________ g simple eye ointment.
- **Theory:** Ophthalmic preparations are sterile products, essentially free from foreign particles, suitably formulated and packaged in suitable container for either topical application to the eyelids or instillation into cul-de-sac between eyeball and eyelid.

  Ophthalmic ointments are ointments meant for application to the eye. It can be used to obtain the effect of a variety of medicaments on the outside and edges of the eyelids. It contains sterilized ingredients packed under rigidly aseptic conditions and meets the requirements of the official sterility tests.

  Eye ointments must be free from large particles and should be prepared with aseptic precautions. For the preparation of simple eye ointment, it is often necessary to vary the proportion of the different ingredients of the bases to maintain a suitable consistency under different climatic conditions. Liquid paraffin, white soft and hard paraffin may be adjusted for this purpose. However, the proportions of the active medicaments must not be altered.

  Uses: Pharmaceutical aid.
- **Procedure:** Melt together weighed amount of wool fat and yellow soft paraffin in a china dish. Add liquid paraffin to make up required weight. Filter the hot mixture through coarse filter paper placed in a heated funnel. Sterilize the filtrate by dry heat at 150°C for sufficient time to ensure that whole is maintained at this temperature for one hour. Allow to cool at room temperature without opening the container.
- **Storage:** 5.0 g in small sterilized collapsible tube with the stated strength should be dispensed unless otherwise directed. Eye ointment may be unstable and should be stored in a cool place.

VIVA VOCE QUESTIONS

Q.1   What are eye ointments?

____

Q.2   Why eye ointments are prepared?

____

Q.3   How will eye ointment be sterilized?

____

Q. 4.   Write the uses of simple eye ointment.

____

❖ ❖ ❖

Formulation Table:

Ingredients	Quantity required for 100 ml	Quantity required for _____ g
Cortisone acetate	2.5 g	_____ g
Polysorbate 80	400 mg	_____ g
Sodium CMC	500 mg	_____ g
Sodium chloride	900 mg	_____ g
Benzyl alcohol	9.0 ml	_____ ml
Purified water	Upto 100 ml	_____ ml

Calculations:

Cortisone acetate required to prepare 100 ml of suspension = 2.5 g

So, for preparation of _____ ml suspension, Cortisone required = $\dfrac{2.5}{100} \times$ —— = —— g

Polysorbate 80 required to prepare 100 ml of suspension = 400 mg = 0.4 g

So, for preparation of _____ ml suspension, Polysorbate required = $\dfrac{0.4}{100} \times$ —— = —— g

Sodium CMC required to prepare 100 ml of suspension = 500 mg = 0.5 g

So, for preparation of _____ ml suspension, Sodium CMC required = $\dfrac{0.5}{100} \times$ —— = —— g

Sodium chloride required to prepare 100 ml of suspension = 900 mg = 0.9 g

So, for preparation of _____ ml suspension, Sodium chloride required = $\dfrac{0.9}{100} \times$ — = — g

Label of Preparation:

CORTISONE ACETATE SUSPENSION			
Each 100 ml contains			
Cortisone acetate : 2.5 g			
Polysorbate 80 : 400 mg			
Sodium CMC : 500 mg			
Sodium chloride : 900 mg			
Benzyl alcohol : 9.0 ml			
Purified water : Upto 100 ml			
Patient Name:		**Age:**	
Sex:		**Weight:**	
Dose: As directed by the physician.			
Mfg. Date:		**Exp. Date:**	
Batch No.:		**Price:**	
Prepared by:			

Date :___________   Marks : _________/10

EXPERIMENT NO. 38

- **Aim:** To prepare ________ ml cortisone acetate suspension.

- **Theory:** A pharmaceutical suspension is a two-phase system in which insoluble solids are dispersed in a liquid medium. The particle size of the dispersed solid is usually greater than 0.5 µm. An aqueous suspension is useful formulation system for administering an insoluble or poorly soluble drug. They are widely administered from various routes. Formulation of suspension contains following additives : Flocculating agents, suspending agents, wetting agents, dispersants, preservatives and organoleptic additives. Suspension is evaluated by its rate of sedimentation, viscosity, particle size, pH, and organoleptic properties.

  Uses: Adrenocortical hormone.

  Dose: 50 to 300 mg by mouth

- **Procedure:** Dissolve all additives in purified water, except cortisone acetate. Disperse and triturate cortisone acetate in the previously mixed additives in glass pestle mortar. Add sufficient purified water to produce 100 ml. Pass dispersion through a colloidal mill.

- **Storage:** Preserve in a well-closed container, and protect from light.

VIVA VOCE QUESTIONS

Q.1   What is suspension?

____

Q.2   Write evaluation of suspensions.

____

Q.3   What are two classes of suspension?

____

❖ ❖ ❖

Formulation Table:

Ingredients	Quantity required for 100 ml	Quantity required for _____ g
Amoxycillin trihydrate	4 g	_____ g
Sodium CMC	1.8 g	_____ g
Colour tartrazine	0.02 g	_____ g
Sodium benzoate	0.45 g	_____ g
Sugar	90.0 g	_____ g
Pineapple flavour	1.0 g	_____ g
Purified water	Upto 100 ml	_____ ml

Calculations:

Amoxycillin trihydrate required to prepare 100 ml of suspension = 4 g

So, for preparation of __ ml suspension, Amoxycillin trihydrate required $= \dfrac{4}{100} \times \text{—} = \text{—} \ g$

Sodium CMC required to prepare 100 ml of suspension = 1.8 g

So, for preparation of _____ ml suspension, Sodium CMC required $= \dfrac{1.8}{100} \times \text{———} = \text{———} \ g$

Sugar required to prepare 100 ml of suspension = 90 g

So, for preparation of _____ ml suspension, sodium chloride required $= \dfrac{90}{100} \times \text{—} = \text{—} \ g$

Label of Preparation:

<table>
<tr><td colspan="4" align="center">AMOXYCILLIN TRIHYDRATE SUSPENSION</td></tr>
<tr><td colspan="4">Each 100 ml contains</td></tr>
<tr><td colspan="4">Amoxycillin trihydrate   : 4 g</td></tr>
<tr><td colspan="4">Sodium CMC   : 1.8 g</td></tr>
<tr><td colspan="4">Colour tartrazine   : 0.02 g</td></tr>
<tr><td colspan="4">Sodium benzoate   : 0.45 g</td></tr>
<tr><td colspan="4">Sugar   : 90.0 g</td></tr>
<tr><td colspan="4">Pineapple flavour   : 1.0 g</td></tr>
<tr><td colspan="4">Purified water   : Upto 100 ml</td></tr>
<tr><td>Patient Name:</td><td></td><td>Age:</td><td></td></tr>
<tr><td>Sex:</td><td></td><td>Weight:</td><td></td></tr>
<tr><td colspan="4">Dose: As directed by the physician.</td></tr>
<tr><td>Mfg. Date:</td><td></td><td>Exp. Date:</td><td></td></tr>
<tr><td>Batch No.:</td><td></td><td>Price:</td><td></td></tr>
<tr><td colspan="4">Prepared by:</td></tr>
</table>

Date :___________   Marks : ________/10

EXPERIMENT NO. 39

- **Aim:** To prepare _________ ml amoxicillin trihydrate suspension.

- **Theory:** A pharmaceutical suspension is a two-phase system in which insoluble solids are dispersed in a liquid medium. The particle size of the dispersed solids is usually greater than 0.5 µm. An aqueous suspension is useful formulation system for administering an insoluble or poorly soluble drug. They are widely administered from various routes. Formulation of suspension contains following additives : Flocculating agents, suspending agents, wetting agents, dispersants, preservatives and organoleptic additives. Suspension is evaluated by its rate of sedimentation, viscosity, particle size, pH, and organoleptic properties.

  Uses: Antibiotic.

  Dose: 250 to 5300 mg by mouth.

- **Procedure:** Dissolve separately colour tartrazine, sodium benzoate and sugar. Mix and add sodium CMC and triturate in pestle mortar. Disperse amoxicillin trihydrate and add flavour. Add sufficient amount of water to produce 100 ml.

- **Storage:** Preserve in a well-closed container and protect from light.

VIVA VOCE QUESTIONS

Q.1   What is suspension?

____

Q.2   Write formulation of suspensions.

____

Q.3   What are evaluations of suspension?

____

❖ ❖ ❖

Formulation Table:

Ingredients	Quantity required for 100 ml	Quantity required for _____ g
Steroid	2.5 g	_____ g
Polysorbate 80	0.2 g	_____ g
Sodium citrate	1.0 g	_____ g
Benzyl alcohol	0.9 ml	_____ ml
Purified water	Upto 100 ml	_____ ml

Calculations:

Steroid required to prepare 100 ml of suspension = 2.5 g

So, for preparation of _____ ml suspension, Steroid required = $\dfrac{2.5}{100} \times$ ——— = ——— g

Polysorbate 80 required to prepare 100 ml of suspension = 0.2 g

So, for preparation of _____ ml suspension, Polysorbate 80 required = $\dfrac{0.2}{100} \times$ ——— = ——— g

Benzyl alcohol required to prepare 100 ml of suspension = 0.9 ml

So, for preparation of _____ ml suspension, Benzyl alcohol required = $\dfrac{0.9}{100} \times$ — = — ml

Label of Preparation:

Steroidal Suspension		
Each 100 ml contains		
Steriod : 2.5 g		
Polysorbate 80 : 0.2 g		
Sodium citrate : 1.0 g		
Benzyl alcohol : 0.9 ml		
Purified water : Upto 100 ml		
Patient Name:		**Age:**	
Sex:		**Weight:**	
Dose: As directed by the physician.			
Mfg. Date:		**Exp. Date:**	
Batch No.:		**Price:**	
Prepared by:			

Date :___________   Marks : ________/10

EXPERIMENT NO. 40

- **Aim:** To prepare ________ ml steroidal suspension.

- **Theory:** A pharmaceutical suspension is a two phase system in which insoluble solids are dispersed in a liquid medium. The particle size of the dispersed solid is usually greater than 0.5 µm. An aqueous suspension is useful formulation system for administering an insoluble or poorly soluble drug. They are widely administered from various routes. Formulation of suspension contains following additives : Flocculating agents, suspending agents, wetting agents, dispersants, preservatives and organoleptic additives. Suspension is evaluated by its rate of sedimentation, viscosity, particle size, pH, and organoleptic properties.

  Uses: Hormone.

  Dose: As directed by physician.

- **Procedure:** Dissolve all additives in purified water except steroid. Disperse steroid. Add sufficient amount of water to produce 100 ml.

- **Storage:** Preserve in a well-closed container and protect from light.

VIVA VOCE QUESTIONS

Q.1   What is the difference between flocculated and deflocculated suspension?

____

Q.2   What is the use of steroidal suspension?

____

Q.3   What are evaluations of suspension?

____

❖ ❖ ❖

Formulation Table:

Ingredients	Quantity required for 100 ml	Quantity required for _____ ml
Liquid paraffin	50.0 ml	_____ ml
Indian gum in powder	12.5 g	_____ g
Tragacanth	0.5 g	_____ g
Sodium benzoate	0.5 g	_____ g
Vanillin	0.005 g	_____ g
Glycerin	12.5 ml	_____ ml
Chloroform	0.25 ml	_____ ml
Purified water	Upto 100 ml	_____ ml

Calculations:

Liquid paraffin required to prepare 100 ml of emulsion = 50 ml

So, for preparation of _____ ml emulsion, Liquid paraffin required = $\dfrac{50}{100} \times$ ——— = ——— ml

Indian gum required to prepare 100 ml of emulsion = 12.5 g

So, for preparation of _____ ml emulsion, Indian gum required = $\dfrac{12.5}{100} \times$ ——— = ——— g

Label of Preparation:

LIQUID PARAFFIN EMULSION		
Each 100 ml contains		
Liquid paraffin	: 50.0 ml	
Indian gum in powder	: 12.5 g	
Tragacanth	: 0.5 g	
Sodium benzoate	: 0.5 g	
Vanillin	: 0.005 g	
Glycerin	: 12.5 ml	
Chloroform	: 0.25 ml	
Purified water	: Upto 100 ml	
Patient Name:		**Age:**
Sex:		**Weight:**
Dose: As directed by the physician.		
Mfg. Date:		**Exp. Date:**
Batch No.:		**Price:**
Prepared by:		

Date :___________   Marks : ________/10

EXPERIMENT NO. 41

- **Aim:** To prepare ________ ml liquid paraffin emulsion.
- **Theory:** Emulsion is a heterogeneous system consisting of at least one immiscible liquid dispersed in another in the form of droplets whose diameter in general exceeds 0.1 µm. Such system possesses a minimal stability because the droplets quickly coalesce and the two liquids get separated. The stability of the emulsion is increased by adding another substance known as emulsifying agent or emulsifier. The liquid droplet is generally known as the emulsion phase or emulsion globules or dispersed phase or internal phase; while the liquid, in which they are dispersed, is known as the continuous phase or dispersion phase.

  Uses: Laxative.

  Dose: 8 to 30 ml.

- **Procedure:** Triturate the weighed quantity of liquid paraffin and chloroform with the Indian gums, tragacanth, and vanillin in mortar and pestle. Add 25.0 ml of purified water and triturate until a creamy emulsion is formed. Dissolve sodium benzoate in small quantity of purified water. Add glycerin and sodium benzoate with continuous triturate. Add sufficient purified water to produce 100 ml of emulsion and mix properly.
- **Storage:** Keep at temperature not exceeding 20°C. Do not refrigerate.

VIVA VOCE QUESTIONS

Q.1   What is emulsion?

____

Q.2   Define laxative, purgative and cathartic effect?

____

Q.3   How to identify type of emulsion?

____

❖ ❖ ❖

Formulation Table:

Ingredients	Quantity required for 100 ml	Quantity required for _____ ml
Castor oil	37.5 ml	_____ ml
Acacia gum powder	10.0 g	_____ g
Cinnamon water sufficient to produce	100 ml	_____ ml

Calculations:

Castor oil required to prepare 100 ml of emulsion = 37.5 ml

So, for preparation of _____ ml emulsion, Castor oil required $= \dfrac{37.5}{100} \times \text{—} = \text{—}$ ml

Acacia gum powder required to prepare 100 ml of emulsion = 10 g

So, for preparation of _____ ml emulsion, Acacia gum powder required

$$= \dfrac{10}{100} \times \text{—} = \text{—} \text{ g}$$

Label of Preparation:

Castor Oil Emulsion			
Each 100 ml contains			
Castor oil	: 37.5 ml		
Acacia gum powder	: 10.0 g		
Cinnamon water	: Upto 100 ml		
Patient Name:		**Age:**	
Sex:		**Weight:**	
Dose: As directed by the physician.			
Mfg. Date:		**Exp. Date:**	
Batch No.:		**Price:**	
Prepared by:			

Date :____________   Marks : ________/10

EXPERIMENT NO. 42

- **Aim:** To prepare ________ ml castor oil emulsion.

- **Theory:** Emulsion is a heterogeneous system consisting of at least one immiscible liquid dispersed in another in the form of droplets whose diameter in general exceeds 0.1 μm. Such system possesses a minimal stability because the droplets quickly coalesce and the two liquids get separated. The stability of the emulsion is increased by adding another substance known as emulsifying agent or emulsifier. The liquid droplet is generally known as the emulsion phase or emulsion globules or dispersed phase or internal phase; while the liquid, in which they are dispersed, is known as the continuous phase or dispersion phase.

  Uses: Laxative.

  Dose: 30 to 60 ml.

- **Procedure:** Triturate the weighed quantity of castor oil and cinnamon water with acacia in mortar and pestle. Add remaining quantity of cinnamon water to produce 100 ml.

- **Storage:** Emulsion should be preserved in a well-closed container.

VIVA VOCE QUESTIONS

Q.1   What is the use of castor oil emulsion?

____

Q.2   Define laxative with examples.

____

Q.3   What is primary emulsion?

____

❖ ❖ ❖

Formulation Table:

Ingredients	Quantity required for 100 ml	Quantity required for _____ ml
Liquid paraffin	25 ml	_______ ml
Chloroform spirit	1.5 ml	_______ ml
Magnesium hydroxide mixture	100 ml	_______ ml

Magnesium hydroxide mixture :

Ingredients	Quantity required for 100 ml	Quantity required for _____ ml
Magnesium sulphate	4.75 g	_______ g
Sodium hydroxide	1.5 g	_______ g
Light magnesium oxide	5.25 g	_______ g
Chloroform	0.25 ml	_______ ml
Purified water sufficient to produce	100 ml	_______ ml

Calculations:

Liquid paraffin required to prepare 100 ml of emulsion = 25 ml

So, for preparation of _____ ml emulsion, Liquid paraffin required = $\dfrac{25}{100} \times$ —— = —— ml

Chloroform spirit required to prepare 100 ml of emulsion = 1.5 ml

So, for preparation of _____ ml emulsion, Chloroform spirit required = $\dfrac{1.5}{100} \times$ —— = —— ml

Label of Preparation:

LIQUID PARAFFIN AND MAGNESIUM HYDROXIDE EMULSION			
Each 100 ml contains			
Liquid paraffin : 25 ml			
Chloroform spirit : 1.5 ml			
Magnesium hydroxide mixture : Upto 100 ml			
Patient Name:		**Age:**	
Sex:		**Weight:**	
Dose: As directed by the physician.			
Mfg. Date:		**Exp. Date:**	
Batch No.:		**Price:**	
Prepared by:			

Date :___________   Marks : _________/10

EXPERIMENT NO. 43

- **Aim:** To prepare _________ ml liquid paraffin and magnesium hydroxide emulsion.
- **Theory:** Emulsion is a heterogeneous system consisting of at least one immiscible liquid dispersed in another in the form of droplets whose diameter in general exceeds 0.1 µm. Such system possesses a minimal stability because the droplets quickly coalesce and the two liquids get separated. The stability of the emulsion is increased by adding another substance known as emulsifying agent or emulsifier. The liquid droplet is generally known as the emulsion phase or emulsion globules or dispersed phase or internal phase; while the liquid, in which they are dispersed, is known as the continuous phase or dispersion phase.

  Uses: Laxative and antacid.

  Dose: 5 to 20 ml.
- **Procedure:** Mix chloroform spirit with 65 ml of magnesium hydroxide mixture. Add liquid paraffin and mix. Add sufficient magnesium hydroxide to produce 100 ml. Pass through homogeniser.
- **Storage:** Store in a well-closed container.

VIVA VOCE QUESTIONS

Q.1   What is the use of liquid paraffin?

____

Q.2   Define antacid?

____

Q.3   What is the use of liquid paraffin and magnesium hydroxide emulsion?

____

❖ ❖ ❖

Formulation Table:

Ingredients	Quantity required for 100 ml	Quantity required for ______ ml
Peppermint oil	2.0 ml	______ ml
Polysorbate-20	0.10 ml	______ ml
Double strength chloroform water	50.0 ml	______ ml
Purified water sufficient to produce	100 ml	______ ml

Calculations:

Peppermint oil required to prepare 100 ml of emulsion = 2.0 ml

So, for preparation of _____ ml emulsion, Liquid paraffin required $= \dfrac{2.0}{100} \times$ ——— $=$ ——— ml

Double strength chloroform water required to prepare 100 ml of emulsion = 50 ml

So, for preparation of ______ ml emulsion, Double strength chloroform required

$$= \dfrac{50}{100} \times \text{———} = \text{———} \ ml$$

Label of Preparation:

PEPPERMINT EMULSION			
Each 100 ml contains			
Peppermint oil	: 2.0 ml		
Polysorbate-20	: 0.10 ml		
Double strength chloroform water	: 50.0 ml		
Purified water	: Up to 100 ml		
Patient Name:		**Age:**	
Sex:		**Weight:**	
Dose: As directed by the physician.			
Mfg. Date:		**Exp. Date:**	
Batch No.:		**Price:**	
Prepared by:			

Date :___________   Marks : _________/10

EXPERIMENT NO. 44

- **Aim:** To prepare _________ ml peppermint emulsion.

- **Theory:** Emulsion is a heterogeneous system consisting of at least one immiscible liquid dispersed in another in the form of droplets whose diameter in general exceeds 0.1 µm. Such system possesses a minimal stability because the droplets quickly coalesce and the two liquids get separated. The stability of the emulsion is increased by adding another substance known as emulsifying agent or emulsifier. The liquid droplet is generally known as the emulsion phase or emulsion globules or dispersed phase or internal phase; while the liquid, in which they are dispersed, is known as the continuous phase or dispersion phase.

  Uses: Carminative.

  Dose: 0.25 to 1.0 ml.

- **Procedure:** Mix peppermint oil with polysorbate-20 by shaking. To this, add double strength chloroform water. Add sufficient purified water to produce 100 ml by shaking.

- **Storage:** Store in a well-closed container.

VIVA VOCE QUESTIONS

Q.1   What is the use of peppermint emulsion?

____

Q.2   How will you prepare peppermint emulsion?

____

Q.3   How will you select emulsifying agent?

____

❖ ❖ ❖

Formulation Table:

Ingredients	Quantity
Bismuth subgallate	200 mg
Resorcinol	60 mg
Zinc oxide	120 mg
Castor oil	60 mg
Theobroma oil, sufficient to fill a mould	q.s.

Label of Preparation:

<table>
<tr><td colspan="4" align="center">BISMUTH SUBGALLATE SUPPOSITORY</td></tr>
<tr><td colspan="4">Each suppository contains</td></tr>
<tr><td colspan="4">Bismuth subgallate   : 200 mg</td></tr>
<tr><td colspan="4">Resorcinol   : 60 mg</td></tr>
<tr><td colspan="4">Zinc oxide   : 120 mg</td></tr>
<tr><td colspan="4">Castor oil   : 60 mg</td></tr>
<tr><td colspan="4">Theobroma oil   : q.s</td></tr>
<tr><td>Patient Name:</td><td></td><td>Age:</td><td></td></tr>
<tr><td>Sex:</td><td></td><td>Weight:</td><td></td></tr>
<tr><td colspan="4">Dose: As directed by the physician.</td></tr>
<tr><td>Mfg. Date:</td><td></td><td>Exp. Date:</td><td></td></tr>
<tr><td>Batch No.:</td><td></td><td>Price:</td><td></td></tr>
<tr><td colspan="4">Prepared by:

</td></tr>
</table>

Date :___________   Marks : _________/10

EXPERIMENT NO. 45

- **Aim:** To prepare compound bismuth subgallate suppositories.

- **Theory:** A suppository is a solid or semi-solid mass meant to be inserted into a body orifice like rectum, vagina and to lesser extent in the urethra to provide either a local or a systemic therapeutic effect. Suppositories can provide systemic effect when used rectally. They are frequently used for local effects for relief of haemorrhoids or infection in the rectum, vagina or urethra.

  Suppositories are mainly of three types:
  (i)   Rectal suppositories,
  (ii) Vaginal suppositories,
  (iii) Urethral suppositories.

  Suppository bases are classified into 3 types:
  (i)   Cocoa butter or theobroma oil,
  (ii) Water soluble or dispersible bases,
  (iii) Glycerinated gelatin

  Uses: Astringent and antacid.

  Dose: 1g.

- **Procedure:** Melt theobroma oil and add other additives. Add remaining amount of theobroma oil and mix uniformly. Properly lubricate the suppository mould. Pour the hot base in the moulds and cool immediately in ice bath. Excess of substance is scrapped off. Open the mould and remove the suppository carefully. Pack in butter paper and store in a well-closed container.

- **Storage:** Stored at a temperature not exceeding 20°C.

VIVA VOCE QUESTIONS

Q.1   What is suppository?

____

Q.2   What are the uses of suppository?

____

Q.3   What are the various types of suppositories?

____

❖❖❖

Formulation Table:

Ingredients	Quantity
Gelatin	14 g
Glycerol	70 g
Purified water, sufficient to produce	q.s.

Label of Preparation:

<table>
<tr><td colspan="4" align="center">GLYCEROL SUPPOSITORY</td></tr>
<tr><td colspan="4">Each suppository contains</td></tr>
<tr><td colspan="4">Gelatin   : 14 g</td></tr>
<tr><td colspan="4">Glycerol   : 70 g</td></tr>
<tr><td colspan="4">Purified water   : q.s.</td></tr>
<tr><td>Patient Name:</td><td></td><td>Age:</td><td></td></tr>
<tr><td>Sex:</td><td></td><td>Weight:</td><td></td></tr>
<tr><td colspan="4">Dose: As directed by the physician.</td></tr>
<tr><td>Mfg. Date:</td><td></td><td>Exp. Date:</td><td></td></tr>
<tr><td>Batch No.:</td><td></td><td>Price:</td><td></td></tr>
<tr><td colspan="4">Prepared by:</td></tr>
</table>

Date :___________   Marks : ________/10

EXPERIMENT NO. 46

- **Aim:** To prepare glycerol suppositories.
- **Theory:** A suppository is a solid or semi-solid mass meant to be inserted into a body orifice like rectum, vagina and to lesser extent in the urethra to provide either a local or a systemic therapeutic effect. Suppositories can provide systemic effect when used rectally. They are frequently used for local effects for relief of haemorrhoids or infection in the rectum, vagina or urethra.

  Suppositories are mainly of three types:

  (i)   Rectal suppositories,

  (ii)   Vaginal suppositories,

  (iii)   Urethral suppositories.

  Suppository bases are classified into three types:

  (i)   Cocoa butter or theobroma oil,

  (ii)   Water soluble or dispersible bases,

  (iii)   Glycerinated gelatin

  Uses: Rectal evacuate.

  Dose: 1 g.

- **Procedure:** Soak gelatin in purified water for about five minutes or until thoroughly softened and then drain well. Add glycerin and heat on water bath. Evaporate excess quantity until the mixture weighs 100 g. Pour the product into suitable moulds.
- **Storage:** Store in a well-closed container, and store in cool place.

VIVA VOCE QUESTIONS

Q.1   What are uses of glycerol suppositories?

____

Q.2   What are the various types of bases?

____

Q.3   What are the various types of suppositories?

____

❖ ❖ ❖

Formulation Table:

Ingredients	Quantity
Gelatin	91 g
Sodium stearate	9 g
Purified water, sufficient to produce	5 g

Label of Preparation:

<table>
<tr><td colspan="4" align="center">GLYCERIN SUPPOSITORY</td></tr>
<tr><td colspan="4">Each suppository contains</td></tr>
<tr><td colspan="4">Gelatin : 91 g</td></tr>
<tr><td colspan="4">Sodium stearate : 9 g</td></tr>
<tr><td colspan="4">Purified water, sufficient to produce : 5 g</td></tr>
<tr><td>Patient Name:</td><td></td><td>Age:</td><td></td></tr>
<tr><td>Sex:</td><td></td><td>Weight:</td><td></td></tr>
<tr><td colspan="4">Dose: As directed by the physician.</td></tr>
<tr><td>Mfg. Date:</td><td></td><td>Exp. Date:</td><td></td></tr>
<tr><td>Batch No.:</td><td></td><td>Price:</td><td></td></tr>
<tr><td colspan="4">Prepared by:

</td></tr>
</table>

Date :___________   Marks : ________/10

EXPERIMENT NO. 47

- **Aim:** To prepare gelatin suppositories.

- **Theory:** A suppository is a solid or semi-solid mass meant to be inserted into a body orifice like rectum, vagina and to lesser extent in the urethra to provide either a local or a systemic therapeutic effect. Suppositories can provide systemic effect when used rectally. They are frequently used for local effects for relief of haemorrhoids or infection in the rectum, vagina or urethra.

  Suppositories are mainly of three types:
  (i)   Rectal suppositories,
  (ii)   Vaginal suppositories,
  (iii) Urethral suppositories.

  Suppository bases are classified into three types:
  (i)   Cocoa butter or theobroma oil,
  (ii)   Water soluble or dispersible bases,
  (iii) Glycerinated gelatin.

  Uses: Local applicant.

- **Procedure:** Heat the weighed amount of glycerin in a suitable container to about 120°C. Dissolve sodium stearate in the heated glycerin with stirring. Add purified water and mix. Pour the hot mixture in suitable mould.

- **Storage:** Store in a well-closed container protected from atmospheric moisture and temperature.

VIVA VOCE QUESTIONS

Q.1   What are the uses of glycerin suppositories?

____

Q.2   What are the various types of bases?

____

Q.3   What are suppositories?

____

❖ ❖ ❖

Formulation Table:

Ingredients	Quantity
Drugs and purified water	10 g
Gelatin	20 g
Glycerin	70 g

Label of Preparation:

GLYCERINATED GELATIN SUPPOSITORY			
Each suppository contains			
Drugs and purified water : 10 g			
Gelatin : 20 g			
Glycerin : 70 g			
Patient Name:		**Age:**	
Sex:		**Weight:**	
Dose: As directed by the physician.			
Mfg. Date:		**Exp. Date:**	
Batch No.:		**Price:**	
Prepared by:			

Date :___________   Marks : _________/10

EXPERIMENT NO. 48

- **Aim:** To prepare glycerinated gelatin suppositories.

- **Theory:** A suppository is a solid or semi-solid mass meant to be inserted into a body orifice like rectum, vagina and to lesser extent in the urethra to provide either a local or a systemic therapeutic effect. Suppositories can provide systemic effect when used rectally. They are frequently used for local effects for relief of haemorrhoids or infection in the rectum, vagina or urethra.

  Suppositories are mainly of three types:

  (i)   Rectal suppositories,
  (ii)   Vaginal suppositories,
  (iii) Urethral suppositories.

  Suppository bases are classified into three types:

  (i)   Cocoa butter or theobroma oil,
  (ii)   Water soluble or dispersible bases,
  (iii) Glycerinated gelatin.

  Uses: Vaginal suppository for local application of antimicrobial agent.

- **Procedure:** Dissolve the drug in purified water. Moisten the gelatin. Heat glycerin and add gelatin and drug solution. Mix uniformly and pour this mixture into mould.

- **Storage:** Store in a well-closed container protected from atmospheric moisture and temperature.

VIVA VOCE QUESTIONS

Q.1   What are the uses of glycerinated gelatin suppositories?

____

Q.2   What is gelatin?

____

Q.3   What are the advantages and disadvantages of suppositories?

____

❖ ❖ ❖

Formulation Table:

Ingredients	Quantity
Tannic acid	0.2 g
Theobroma oil	q.s.

Label of Preparation:

<table>
<tr><td colspan="4" align="center">TANNIC ACID SUPPOSITORY</td></tr>
<tr><td colspan="4">Each suppository contains</td></tr>
<tr><td colspan="4">Tannic acid   :   0.2 g</td></tr>
<tr><td colspan="4">Theobroma oil   :   q.s.</td></tr>
<tr><td>Patient Name:</td><td></td><td>Age:</td><td></td></tr>
<tr><td>Sex:</td><td></td><td>Weight:</td><td></td></tr>
<tr><td colspan="4">Dose: As directed by the physician.</td></tr>
<tr><td>Mfg. Date:</td><td></td><td>Exp. Date:</td><td></td></tr>
<tr><td>Batch No.:</td><td></td><td>Price:</td><td></td></tr>
<tr><td colspan="4">Prepared by:</td></tr>
</table>

Date :___________   Marks : _________/10

EXPERIMENT NO. 49

- **Aim:** To prepare tannic acid suppositories.
- **Theory:** A suppository is a solid or semi-solid mass meant to be inserted into a body orifice like rectum, vagina and to lesser extent in the urethra to provide either a local or a systemic therapeutic effect. Suppositories can provide systemic effect when used rectally. They are frequently used for local effects for relief of haemorrhoids or infection in the rectum, vagina or urethra.

  Suppositories are mainly of three types:
  (i)   Rectal suppositories,
  (ii) Vaginal suppositories,
  (iii) Urethral suppositories.

  Suppository bases are classified into three types:
  (i)   Cocoa butter or theobroma oil,
  (ii) Water soluble or dispersible bases,
  (iii) Glycerinated gelatin.

  Uses: Astringent.
- **Procedure:** Add lubricant in mould and remove the excess of lubricant by draining. Cool the lubricated mould over ice. Heat theobroma oil in porcelain dish over a water bath and avoid overheating. Remove dish from water bath as soon as the mass is molten. Powder the weighed amount of tannic acid. Add powdered tannic acid in molten theobroma oil. Mix the tannic acid by spatula (sometimes molten theobroma oil is divided into two parts), until it is sufficiently thickened and flows sluggishly and then pour the mixture into the mould. Fill each mould and stir the contents of the dishes during the pouring. Place the mould on ice and remove the excess mass carefully by sharp knife. When suppositories have set hard, open the mould and remove the suppositories by slight pressure on broad ends. Remove the lubricant on final product, by rolling on the filter paper.
- **Storage:** Should be stored in a well-closed tight container.

VIVA VOCE QUESTIONS

Q.1   What are the uses of tannic acid suppositories?

Q.2   What is theobroma oil?

Q.3   What are astringents?

❖❖❖

Formulation Table:

Ingredients	Quantity required for 15 ml	Quantity required for _____ ml
Aluminum sulphate	4.5 g	_______ g
Acetic acid	5.0 ml	_______ ml
Tartaric acid	0.9 g	_______ g
Calcium carbonate	2.0 g	_______ g
Purified water upto	15.0 ml	_______ ml

Calculations:

Aluminium sulphate required to prepare 15 ml of ear drops = 4.5 g

So, for preparation of _____ ml ear drops, Aluminium sulphate required = $\dfrac{4.5}{15} \times \text{---} = \text{---}$ g

Acetic acid required to prepare 15 ml of ear drops = 5.0 ml

So, for preparation of _____ ml ear drops, Acetic acid required = $\dfrac{5.0}{15} \times \text{-----} = \text{-----}$ ml

Tartaric acid required to prepare 15 ml of ear drops = 0.9 g

So, for preparation of _____ ml ear drops, Tartaric acid required = $\dfrac{0.9}{15} \times \text{-----} = \text{-----}$ g

Calcium carbonate required to prepare 15 ml of ear drops = 2.0 g

So, for preparation of _____ ml ear drops, Calcium carbonate required = $\dfrac{2.0}{15} \times \text{---} = \text{---}$ g

Label of Preparation:

ALUMINIUM ACETATE EAR DROP			
Each 15 ml contains			
Aluminum sulphate : 4.5 g			
Acetic acid : 5.0 ml			
Tartaric acid : 0.9 g			
Calcium carbonate : 2.0 g			
Purified water : 15.0 ml			
Patient Name:		**Age:**	
Sex:		**Weight:**	
Dose: As directed by the physician.			
Mfg. Date:		**Exp. Date:**	
Batch No.:		**Price:**	
Prepared by:			

Date :___________   Marks : ________/10

EXPERIMENT NO. 50

- **Aim:** To prepare ________ ml aluminium acetate ear drops.

- **Theory:** Ear drops are liquid preparations and usually are suspensions or emulsions or solutions consisting of one or more active ingredients. Ear drops are generally safe for the ears even if there is damage in ear drum. Ear drops are generally gentle enough for the middle air. The ingredients of ear drops are different depending on the purpose. 15 ml of ear drops should be dispensed unless and otherwise directed. Ear drops are designed to soften the ear wax and to cure bacterial fungus.

  Uses: Astringent and as a local antiperspirant.

  Dose: 3 to 5 drops.

- **Procedure:** Weigh required amount of aluminium sulphate and dissolve in 10 ml of purified water. Add acetic acid and then calcium carbonate. Add remaining amount of purified water and mix properly. Allow to stand for not less than 24 hours in a cool place. Filter the solution and add tartaric acid in the filtrate.

VIVA VOCE QUESTIONS

Q.1   Why ear drops are required?

____

Q.2   What is the difference between ear drops and eye drops?

____

Q.3   How will you prepare ear drops?

____

❖ ❖ ❖

Formulation Table:

Ingredients	Quantity required for 10 ml	Quantity required for _____ ml
Sodium bicarbonate	0.75 g	_____ g
Glycerin	4.5 ml	_____ ml
Purified water upto	10.0 ml	_____ ml

Calculations:

Sodium bicarbonate required to prepare 10 ml of ear drops = 0.75 g

So, for preparation of ____ ml ear drops, Sodium bicarbonate required = $\dfrac{0.75}{10} \times -\!- = -\!-$ g

Glycerin required to prepare 10 ml of ear drops = 4.5 ml

So, for preparation of _____ ml ear drops, Glycerin required = $\dfrac{4.5}{10} \times -\!- = -\!-$ ml

Label of Preparation:

SODIUM BICARBONATE EAR DROP			
Each 10 ml contains			
Sodium bicarbonate : 0.75 g			
Glycerin : 4.5 ml			
Purified water : 15.0 ml			
Patient Name:		**Age:**	
Sex:		**Weight:**	
Dose: As directed by the physician.			
Mfg. Date:		**Exp. Date:**	
Batch No.:		**Price:**	
Prepared by:			

Date :___________ Marks : ________/10

EXPERIMENT NO. 51

- **Aim:** To prepare ________ ml sodium bicarbonate ear drops.

- **Theory:** Ear drops are liquid preparations and usually are suspensions or emulsions or solutions consisting of one or more active ingredients. Ear drops are generally safe for the ears even if there is damage in ear drum. Ear drops are generally gentle enough for the middle air. The ingredients of ear drops are different depending on the purpose. Generally 15 ml of ear drops are to be dispensed unless and otherwise directed. Ear drops are designed to soften the ear wax and to cure bacterial fungus.

  Uses: Antipruritic.

  Dose: 3 to 5 drops.

- **Procedure:** Dissolve sodium bicarbonate in freshly boiled and cooled water in about 6 ml. Add glycerin and mix. Add sufficient purified water to produce 10.0 ml.

VIVA VOCE QUESTIONS

Q.1   What is the use of sodium bicarbonate ear drops?

____

Q.2   How will you prepare ear drops?

____

Q.3   What is the use of glycerin in ear drops?

____

❖ ❖ ❖

Formulation Table:

Ingredients	Quantity required for 15 ml	Quantity required for _____ ml
Hydrogen peroxide	3.75 ml	_______ ml
Purified water upto	15.0 ml	_______ ml

Calculations:

Hydrogen peroxide required to prepare 15 ml of ear drops = 3.75 ml

So, for preparation of ____ ml ear drops, Hydrogen peroxide required

$$= \frac{3.75}{15} \times \text{------} = \text{------ ml}$$

Label of Preparation:

HYDROGEN PEROXIDE EAR DROPS			
Each 15 ml contains			
Hydrogen peroxide : 3.75 ml			
Purified water upto : 15.0 ml			
Patient Name:		**Age:**	
Sex:		**Weight:**	
Dose: As directed by the physician.			
Mfg. Date:		**Exp. Date:**	
Batch No.:		**Price:**	
Prepared by:			

Date :___________   Marks : ________/10

EXPERIMENT NO. 52

- **Aim:** To prepare ________ ml hydrogen peroxide ear drops.

- **Theory:** Ear drops are liquid preparations and usually are suspensions or emulsions or solutions consisting of one or more active ingredients. Ear drops are generally safe for the ears even if there is damage in ear drum. Ear drops are generally gentle enough for the middle air. The ingredients of ear drops are different depending on the purpose. Generally 15 ml of ear drops are to be dispensed unless and otherwise directed. Ear drops are designed to soften the ear wax and to cure bacterial fungus.

  Uses: Softens ear wax solution.

  Dose: 3 to 5 drops.

- **Procedure:** Mix measured amount of hydrogen peroxide solution with purified water. If any turbidity or impurity persists, filter the solution.

VIVA VOCE QUESTIONS

Q.1   What is hydrogen peroxide?

____

Q.2   What is the use of hydrogen peroxide ear drops?

____

Q.3   Whether ear drops are external preparation or internal preparation?

____

❖ ❖ ❖

Formulation Table:

Ingredients	Quantity required for 15 ml	Quantity required for _____ ml
Boric acid	0.2 g	_____ g
Denatured spirit	3.0 ml	_____ ml
Purified water upto	15.0 ml	_____ ml

Calculations:

Boric acid required to prepare 15 ml of ear drops = 0.2 g

So, for preparation of _____ ml ear drops, Boric acid required = $\dfrac{0.2}{15} \times$ ——— = ——— g

Denatured spirit required to prepare 15 ml of ear drops = 3.0 ml

So, for preparation of _____ ml ear drops, Boric acid required = $\dfrac{3.0}{15} \times$ ——— = ——— ml

Label of Preparation:

<table>
<tr><td colspan="4" align="center">BORIC ACID EAR DROPS</td></tr>
<tr><td colspan="4">Each 15 ml contains</td></tr>
<tr><td colspan="4">Boric acid   :   0.2 g
Denatured spirit   :   3.0 ml
Purified water upto   :   15.0 ml</td></tr>
<tr><td>Patient Name:</td><td></td><td>Age:</td><td></td></tr>
<tr><td>Sex:</td><td></td><td>Weight:</td><td></td></tr>
<tr><td colspan="4">Dose: As directed by the physician.</td></tr>
<tr><td>Mfg. Date:</td><td></td><td>Exp. Date:</td><td></td></tr>
<tr><td>Batch No.:</td><td></td><td>Price:</td><td></td></tr>
<tr><td colspan="4">Prepared by:

 </td></tr>
</table>

Date :___________   Marks : ________/10

EXPERIMENT NO. 53

- **Aim:** To prepare _______ ml boric acid ear drops.

- **Theory:** Ear drops are liquid preparations and usually are suspensions or emulsions or solutions consisting of one or more active ingredients. Ear drops are generally safe for the ears even if there is damage in ear drum. Ear drops are generally gentle enough for the middle air. The ingredients of ear drops are different depending on the purpose. Generally 15 ml of ear drops are to be dispensed unless and otherwise directed. Ear drops are designed to soften the ear wax and to cure bacterial fungus.

  Uses: Local anti-infective.

  Dose: 3 to 5 drops.

- **Procedure:** Dissolve weighed quantity of boric acid in denatured spirit. Add purified water and make sufficient volume to produce 15.0 ml. If any impurities are present, then filter it and dispense it in a suitable container.

VIVA VOCE QUESTIONS

Q.1   What is boric acid?

____

Q.2   What is the use of boric acid ear drops?

____

Q.3   What are germicides? Give example.

____

❖ ❖ ❖

Formulation Table:

Ingredients	Quantity required for 15 ml	Quantity required for _____ ml
Chloramphenicol	0.75 g	_______ g
Propylene glycol upto	15.0 ml	_______ ml

Calculations:

Chloramphenicol required to prepare 15 ml of ear drops = 0.75 g

So, for preparation of _____ ml ear drops, Chloramphenicol required

$$= \frac{0.75}{15} \times \text{——} = \text{——} \text{ g}$$

Label of Preparation:

CHLORAMPHENICOL EAR DROPS			
Each 15 ml contains			
Chloramphenicol : 0.75 g			
Propylene glycol upto : 15.0 ml			
Patient Name:		**Age:**	
Sex:		**Weight:**	
Dose: As directed by the physician.			
Mfg. Date:		**Exp. Date:**	
Batch No.:		**Price:**	
Prepared by:			

Date :______________   Marks : ________/10

EXPERIMENT NO. 54

- **Aim:** To prepare ________ ml chloramphenicol ear drops.

- **Theory:** Ear drops are liquid preparations and usually are suspensions or emulsions or solutions consisting of one or more active ingredients. Ear drops are generally safe for the ears even if there is damage in ear drum. Ear drops are generally gentle enough for the middle air. The ingredients of ear drops are different depending on the purpose. Generally 15 ml of ear drops are to be dispensed unless and otherwise directed. Ear drops are designed to soften the ear wax and to cure bacterial fungus.

  Uses: Antibiotic.

  Dose: 3 to 5 drops.

- **Procedure:** Dissolve chloramphenicol in propylene glycol. Shake and add remaining quantity of propylene glycol to produce sufficient volume of 15 ml.

- **Storage:** Preserve in a well-closed container and protect from light and contamination.

VIVA VOCE QUESTIONS

Q.1   What is antibiotic?

____

Q.2   What is the difference between broad spectrum and narrow spectrum antibiotics?

____

Q.3   What are the storage conditions for ear drops?

____

❖ ❖ ❖

Formulation Table:

Ingredients	Quantity required for 15 ml	Quantity required for _____ ml
Framycetin sulphate	0.3 g	_____ g
Water for injection	0.6 ml	_____ ml
Glycerin upto	15.0 ml	_____ ml

Calculations:

Framycetin sulphate required to prepare 15 ml of ear drops = 0.3 g

So, for preparation of _____ ml ear drops, Framycetin sulphate required = $\dfrac{0.3}{15} \times$ —— = — g

Water required to prepare 15 ml of ear drops = 0.6 ml

So, for preparation of _____ ml ear drops, water required = $\dfrac{0.6}{15} \times$ —— = —— ml

Label of Preparation:

FARMYCETIN EAR DROPS		
Each 15 ml contains		
Framycetin sulphate : 0.3 g		
Water for injection : 0.6 ml		
Glycerin upto : 15.0 ml		
Patient Name:	**Age:**	
Sex:	**Weight:**	
Dose: As directed by the physician.		
Mfg. Date:	**Exp. Date:**	
Batch No.:	**Price:**	
Prepared by:		

Date :___________   Marks : ________/10

EXPERIMENT NO. 55

- **Aim:** To prepare ________ ml framycetin ear drops.

- **Theory:** Ear drops are liquid preparations and usually are suspensions or emulsions or solutions consisting of one or more active ingredients. Ear drops are generally safe for the ears even if there is damage in ear drum. Ear drops are generally gentle enough for the middle air. The ingredients of ear drops are different depending on the purpose. Generally 15 ml of ear drops are to be dispensed unless and otherwise directed. Ear drops are designed to soften the ear wax and to cure bacterial fungus.

  Uses: Antibiotic.

  Dose: 3 to 5 drops.

- **Procedure:** Dissolve framycetin sulphate in glycerin with water for injection. Add sterilized glycerin to produce 15 ml.

- **Storage:** Preserve in a well-closed container and protect from light and contamination.

VIVA VOCE QUESTIONS

Q.1   What is framycetin?

____

Q.2   How will you prepare framycetin ear drops?

____

Q.3   What are storage conditions for ear drops?

____

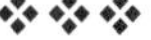

Formulation Table:

Ingredients	Quantity required for 15 ml	Quantity required for _____ ml
Ichthammol	1.5 g	_____ g
Glycerin upto	15.0 ml	_____ ml

Calculations:

Ichthammol required to prepare 15 ml of ear drops = 1.5 g

So, for preparation of _____ ml ear drops, Ichthammol required $= \dfrac{1.5}{15} \times \underline{\hspace{1cm}} = \underline{\hspace{1cm}}$ g

Label of Preparation:

ICHTHAMMOL EAR DROPS			
Each 15 ml contains			
Ichthammol : 1.5 g			
Glycerin upto : 15.0 ml			
Patient Name:		**Age:**	
Sex:		**Weight:**	
Dose: As directed by the physician.			
Mfg. Date:		**Exp. Date:**	
Batch No.:		**Price:**	
Prepared by:			

Date :____________   Marks : _________/10

EXPERIMENT NO. 56

- **Aim:** To prepare _________ ml ichthammol ear drops.

- **Theory:** Ear drops are liquid preparations and usually are suspensions or emulsions or solutions consisting of one or more active ingredients. Ear drops are generally safe for the ears even if there is damage in ear drum. Ear drops are generally gentle enough for the middle air. The ingredients of ear drops are different depending on the purpose. Generally 15 ml of ear drops are to be dispensed unless and otherwise directed. Ear drops are designed to soften the ear wax and to cure bacterial fungus.

  Uses: Antiparasitic.

  Dose: 3 to 5 drops.

- **Procedure:** Dissolve ichthammol in glycerin and filter. Add sterilized glycerin to produce 15 ml.

- **Storage:** Preserve in a well-closed container and protect from light and contamination.

VIVA VOCE QUESTIONS

Q.1   What is Ichthammol?

____

Q.2   How will you prepare this ear drops?

____

Q.3   What is antiparasitic?

____

❖ ❖ ❖

Formulation Table:

Ingredients	Quantity required for 15 ml	Quantity required for _____ ml
Phenol glycerin	6.0 ml	_______ ml
Glycerin upto	15.0 ml	_______ ml

Calculations:

Phenol glycerin required to prepare 15 ml of ear drops = 6.0 ml

So, for preparation of _____ ml ear drops, Phenol glycerin required

$$= \frac{6.0}{15} \times \underline{\qquad} = \underline{\qquad} \text{ ml}$$

Label of Preparation:

PHENOL GLYCERINE EAR DROPS			
Each 15 ml contains			
Phenol glycerin　　　:　6.0 ml			
Glycerin upto　　　　:　15.0 ml			
Patient Name:		**Age:**	
Sex:		**Weight:**	
Dose: As directed by the physician.			
Mfg. Date:		**Exp. Date:**	
Batch No.:		**Price:**	
Prepared by:			

Date :___________   Marks : ________/10

EXPERIMENT NO. 57

- **Aim:** To prepare ________ ml phenol glycerin ear drops.
- **Theory:** Ear drops are liquid preparations and usually are suspensions or emulsions or solutions consisting of one or more active ingredients. Ear drops are generally safe for the ears even if there is damage in ear drum. Ear drops are generally gentle enough for the middle air. The ingredients of ear drops are different depending on the purpose. Generally 15 ml of ear drops are to be dispensed unless and otherwise directed. Ear drops are designed to soften the ear wax and to cure bacterial fungus.

  Uses: Disinfectant.

  Dose: 3 to 5 drops.

- **Procedure:** Mix phenol glycerin with glycerin and shake it. Add glycerin in sufficient amount to produce 15 ml.
- **Storage:** Preserve in a well-closed container and protect from light and contamination.

VIVA VOCE QUESTIONS

Q.1   What is the use of phenol glycerin?

____

Q.2   Why glycerin is used in this preparation?

____

Q.3   What is disinfectant?

____

❖❖❖

Formulation Table:

Ingredients	Quantity required for 15 ml	Quantity required for _____ ml
Magnesium sulphate	1.5 g	_____ g
Purified water	6.0 ml	_____ ml
Glycerin upto	15.0 ml	_____ ml

Calculations:

Magnesium sulphate required to prepare 15 ml of ear drops = 1.5 g

So, for preparation of ____ ml ear drops, Magnesium sulphate required

$$= \frac{1.5}{15} \times \text{——} = \text{——} \; g$$

Purified water required to prepare 15 ml of ear drops = 6.0 ml

So, for preparation of _____ ml ear drops, Purified water required $= \dfrac{6.0}{15} \times \text{——} = \text{——} \; ml$

Label of Preparation:

<table>
<tr><td colspan="3" align="center">MAGNESIUM SULPHATE GLYCERINE EAR DROPS</td></tr>
<tr><td colspan="3">Each 15 ml contains</td></tr>
<tr><td colspan="3">Magnesium sulphate   :   1.5 g</td></tr>
<tr><td colspan="3">Purified water   :   6.0 ml</td></tr>
<tr><td colspan="3">Glycerin upto   :   15.0 ml</td></tr>
<tr><td>Patient Name:</td><td>Age:</td><td></td></tr>
<tr><td>Sex:</td><td>Weight:</td><td></td></tr>
<tr><td colspan="3">Dose: As directed by the physician.</td></tr>
<tr><td>Mfg. Date:</td><td>Exp. Date:</td><td></td></tr>
<tr><td>Batch No.:</td><td>Price:</td><td></td></tr>
<tr><td colspan="3">Prepared by:</td></tr>
</table>

Date :___________   Marks : _________/10

EXPERIMENT NO. 58

- **Aim:** To prepare ________ ml magnesium sulphate glycerin ear drops.
- **Theory:** Ear drops are liquid preparations and usually are suspensions or emulsions or solutions consisting of one or more active ingredients. Ear drops are generally safe for the ears even if there is damage in ear drum. Ear drops are generally gentle enough for the middle air. The ingredients of ear drops are different depending on the purpose. Generally 15 ml of ear drops are to be dispensed unless and otherwise directed. Ear drops are designed to soften the ear wax and to cure bacterial fungus.

  Uses: Ear wax softener.

  Dose: 3 to 5 drops.
- **Procedure:** Dissolve magnesium sulphate in purified water. Add glycerin in sufficient amount to produce 15 ml.
- **Storage:** Preserve in a well-closed container and protect from light and contamination.

VIVA VOCE QUESTIONS

Q.1   What is the use of magnesium sulphate?

____

Q.2   How does it soften the ear wax?

____

Q.3   What is ear wax?

____

❖ ❖ ❖

Formulation Table:

Ingredients	Quantity required for 15 ml	Quantity required for _____ ml
Salicylic acid	0.12 g	_____ g
Glycerin	8.0 ml	_____ ml
Denatured spirit upto	15.0 ml	_____ ml

Calculations:

Salicylic acid required to prepare 15 ml of ear drops = 0.12 g

So, for preparation of _____ ml ear drops, Salicylic acid required = $\dfrac{0.12}{15}$ × —— = —— g

Glycerin required to prepare 15 ml of ear drops = 8.0 ml

So, for preparation of _____ ml ear drops, Glycerin required = $\dfrac{8.0}{15}$ × —— = —— ml

Label of Preparation:

SALICYLIC ACID EAR DROP			
Each 15 ml contains			
Salicylic acid : 0.12 g			
Glycerin : 8.0 ml			
Denatured spirit upto : 15.0 ml			
Patient Name:		**Age:**	
Sex:		**Weight:**	
Dose: As directed by the physician.			
Mfg. Date:		**Exp. Date:**	
Batch No.:		**Price:**	
Prepared by:			

Date :___________   Marks : _________/10

EXPERIMENT NO. 59

- **Aim:** To prepare _______ ml salicylic acid ear drops.
- **Theory:** Ear drops are liquid preparations and usually are suspensions or emulsions or solutions consisting of one or more active ingredients. Ear drops are generally safe for the ears even if there is damage in ear drum. Ear drops are generally gentle enough for the middle air. The ingredients of ear drops are different depending on the purpose. Generally 15 ml of ear drops are to be dispensed unless and otherwise directed. Ear drops are designed to soften the ear wax and to cure bacterial fungus.

  Uses: Analgesic.

  Dose: 3 to 5 drops.
- **Procedure:** Dissolve weighed amount of salicylic acid in denatured spirit. Add glycerin with shaking. Add purified water to produce 15 ml.
- **Storage:** Preserve in a well-closed container and protect from light and contamination.

VIVA VOCE QUESTIONS

Q.1   How will you prepare salicylic acid ear drops?

____

Q.2   What are the storage conditions of ear drops?

____

Q.3   What are analgesics?

____

❖ ❖ ❖

Formulation Table:

Ingredients	Quantity required for 100 ml	Quantity required for _____ ml
Sucrose	66.7 g	_______ g
Water QS	100 g	_______ g

Calculations:

Sucrose required to prepare 100 ml of syrup = 66.7 g

So, for preparation of _____ ml syrup, Sucrose required = $\dfrac{66.7}{100}$ × —— = —— g

Label of Preparation:

SIMPLE SYRUP			
Each 100 ml contains			
Sucrose : 66.7 g Water : 100 g			
Patient Name:		**Age:**	
Sex:		**Weight:**	
Dose: As directed by the physician.			
Mfg. Date:		**Exp. Date:**	
Batch No.:		**Price:**	
Prepared by:			

Date :___________   Marks : _________/10

EXPERIMENT NO. 60

- **Aim:** To prepare _________ ml simple syrup.

- **Theory:** Syrups are concentrated oral solutions of sugar or nearly saturated solutions of sucrose in water. 65% w/w syrups retard the growth of micro-organisms. It is important to note that sucrose concentration should not reach the saturation point, as a saturated solution may lead to crystallization of sucrose. Syrups are classified into the classes like simple syrups, medicated syrups, flavoured syrups.

  Category: Pharmaceutical aid.

- **Procedure:** Transfer the weighed amount of sucrose in a conical flask. Add sufficient amount of water. Make the syrup by heating or without heating. Macerate it with cold water or heat the solution. It can also be agitated to accelerate the solubilisation. Filter the syrup, if necessary. Store in dark container in cool place.

- **Storage:** Store in a cool place.

VIVA VOCE QUESTIONS

Q.1   What is syrup?

____

Q.2   What is fermentation?

____

Q.3   How does syrup act as a self preservative?

____

❖ ❖ ❖

Formulation Table:

Invert syrup (A)

Ingredients	Quantity required for 100 ml	Quantity required for _____ ml
Lemon Spirit	0.5 ml	_____ ml
Citric acid monohydrate	2.5 g	_____ g
Invert syrup	10.0 ml	_____ ml
Syrup QS	100.0 ml	_____ ml

Lemon Spirit (B)

Ingredients	Quantity required for 100 ml	Quantity required for _____ ml
Lemon oil	10.0 ml	_____ ml
Ethyl alcohol	90.0 ml	_____ ml

Label of Preparation:

LEMON SYRUP			
Each 100 ml contains			
Lemon Spirit	: 0.5 ml		
Citric acid monohydrate	: 2.5 g		
Invert syrup	: 10.0 ml		
Syrup QS	: 100.0		
Patient Name:		**Age:**	
Sex:		**Weight:**	
Dose: As directed by the physician.			
Mfg. Date:		**Exp. Date:**	
Batch No.:		**Price:**	
Prepared by:			

Date :___________   Marks : _________/10

EXPERIMENT NO. 61

- **Aim:** To prepare _______ ml lemon syrup.

- **Theory:** Syrups are concentrated oral solutions of sugar or nearly saturated solutions of sucrose in water. 65% w/w syrups retard the growth of micro-organisms. It is important to note that sucrose concentration should not reach the saturation point, as a saturated solution may lead to crystallization of sucrose. Syrups are classified into the classes like simple syrups, medicated syrups, flavoured syrups.

  Category: Pharmaceutical aid.

- **Procedure:** Cut the slices of lemon and prepare lemon spirit by maceration process using 80% alcohol. Dissolve citric acid monohydrate in simple syrup. Add freshly prepared invert syrup and lemon spirit, prepared using formula A & B. Mix it properly. Add sufficient syrup to produce 100 ml.

- **Storage:** Store in a cool place.

VIVA VOCE QUESTIONS

Q.1   What is syrup?

____

Q.2   What is fermentation?

____

Q.3   How does syrup act as a self preservative?

____

❖ ❖ ❖

Formulation Table:

Ingredients	Quantity required for 100 ml	Quantity required for _____ ml
Orange tincture	6.0 g	_____ g
Syrup QS	100.0 ml	_____ ml

Orange Tincture

Ingredients	Quantity required for 100 ml	Quantity required for _____ ml
Fresh orange peel	85.0 g	_____ g
Ethyl alcohol	100.0 ml	_____ ml

Label of Preparation:

ORANGE SYRUP		
Each 100 ml contains		
Fresh orange peel : 85.0 g		
Syrup QS : 100.0 ml		
Patient Name:		**Age:**
Sex:		**Weight:**
Dose: As directed by the physician.		
Mfg. Date:		**Exp. Date:**
Batch No.:		**Price:**
Prepared by:		

Date :___________   Marks : ________/10

EXPERIMENT NO. 62

- **Aim:** To prepare _________ ml orange syrup.

- **Theory:** Syrups are concentrated oral solutions of sugar or nearly saturated solutions of sucrose in water. 65% w/w syrups retard the growth of micro-organisms. It is important to note that sucrose concentration should not reach the saturation point, as a saturated solution may lead to crystallization of sucrose. Syrups are classified into the classes like simple syrups, medicated syrups, flavoured syrups.

  Category: Pharmaceutical aid.

- **Procedure:** Prepare orange tincture by the maceration process. Mix the orange tincture with syrup and make up the volume.

- **Storage:** Store in a cool place.

VIVA VOCE QUESTIONS

Q.1   What is orange syrup?

____

Q.2   What is the use of orange syrup?

____

Q.3   How to prepare orange tincture?

____

❖ ❖ ❖

Formulation Table:

Ingredients	Quantity required for 100 ml	Quantity required for _____ ml
Vasaka liquid extract	50.0 ml	_____ ml
Glycerin	10.0 ml	_____ ml
Syrup QS	100.0 ml	_____ ml

Vasaka Liquid Extract

Ingredients	Quantity required for 100 ml	Quantity required for _____ ml
Vasaka powder	100.0 g	_____ g
Ethyl alcohol	100.0 ml	_____ ml

Label of Preparation:

VASAKA SYRUP			
Each 100 ml contains			
Vasaka liquid extract : 50.0 ml			
Glycerin : 10.0 ml			
Syrup QS : 100.0 ml			
Patient Name:		**Age:**	
Sex:		**Weight:**	
Dose: As directed by the physician.			
Mfg. Date:		**Exp. Date:**	
Batch No.:		**Price:**	
Prepared by:			

Date :___________   Marks : _________/10

EXPERIMENT NO. 63

- **Aim:** To prepare _________ ml vasaka syrup.

- **Theory:** Syrups are concentrated oral solutions of sugar or nearly saturated solutions of sucrose in water. 65% w/w syrups retard the growth of microorganisms. It is important to note that sucrose concentration should not reach the saturation point, as a saturated solution may lead to crystallization of sucrose. Syrups are classified into the classes like simple syrups, medicated syrups, flavoured syrups.

  Category: Expectorant.

  Dose: 2 to 4 ml.

- **Procedure:** Prepare vasaka liquid extract by percolation process. Mix vasaka liquid extract with measured amount of glycerin and shake thoroughly. Add sufficient quantity of syrup and mix properly. Store in a suitable container and put label properly.

- **Storage:** Store in a cool place.

VIVA VOCE QUESTIONS

Q.1   What is source of vasaka?

____

Q.2   What is the use of vasaka syrup?

____

Q.3   What is the dose of vaska syrup?

____

❖ ❖ ❖

Formulation Table:

Ingredients	Quantity required for 100 ml	Quantity required for _____ ml
Strong ginger tincture	5.0 ml	_____ ml
Syrup QS	100.0 ml	_____ ml

Strong Ginger Tincture:

Ingredients	Quantity required for 100 ml	Quantity required for _____ ml
Coarse ginger powder	50.0 g	_____ g
Ethyl alcohol	100.0 ml	_____ ml

Label of Preparation:

GINGER SYRUP			
Each 100 ml contains			
Strong ginger tincture : 5.0 ml			
Syrup QS : 100.0 ml			
Patient Name:		**Age:**	
Sex:		**Weight:**	
Dose: As directed by the physician.			
Mfg. Date:		**Exp. Date:**	
Batch No.:		**Price:**	
Prepared by:			

Date :___________   Marks : ________/10

EXPERIMENT NO. 64

- **Aim:** To prepare ________ ml ginger syrup.
- **Theory:** Syrups are concentrated oral solutions of sugar or nearly saturated solutions of sucrose in water. 65% w/w syrups retard the growth of microorganisms. It is important to note that sucrose concentration should not reach the saturation point, as a saturated solution may lead to crystallization of sucrose. Syrups are classified into the classes like simple syrups, medicated syrups, flavoured syrups.

  Ginger is the rhizome of *Zingiber officianale* scraped to remove the dark outer skin and dried in the sun light. It is used as flavouring agent, intestinal stimulant and carminative in colic and in diarrhoea.

  Category: Carminative.

  Dose: 2 to 4 ml.

- **Procedure:** Prepare strong ginger tincture by percolation process. Add sufficient quantity of syrup and mix properly. Store in a suitable container and put label properly.
- **Storage:** Preserve in a well-closed container.

VIVA VOCE QUESTIONS

Q.1   What is source of ginger?

____

Q.2   Which part of ginger is used in medicine?

____

Q.3   What is the use if ginger syrup?

____

❖ ❖ ❖

Formulation Table:

Ingredients	Quantity required for 100 ml	Quantity required for _____ ml
Codeine phosphate	0.5 g	_____ g
Chloroform spirit	2.5 ml	_____ ml
Purified water	1.5 ml	_____ ml
Syrup QS	100.0 ml	_____ ml

Calculations:

Codeine phosphate required to prepare 100 ml of syrup =   0.5 g

So, for preparation of _____ ml syrup, Codeine phosphate required $= \dfrac{0.5}{100} \times \text{——} = \text{——} \; g$

Chloroform spirit required to prepare 100 ml of syrup = 2.5 ml

So, for preparation of _____ ml syrup, Chloroform spirit required $= \dfrac{2.5}{100} \times \text{——} = \text{——} \; ml$

Label of Preparation:

<table>
<tr><td colspan="4" align="center">CODEINE PHOSPHATE SYRUP</td></tr>
<tr><td colspan="4">Each 100 ml contains</td></tr>
<tr><td colspan="4">Codeine phosphate　　:　0.5 g</td></tr>
<tr><td colspan="4">Chloroform spirit　　:　2.5 ml</td></tr>
<tr><td colspan="4">Purified water　　:　1.5 ml</td></tr>
<tr><td colspan="4">Syrup QS　　:　100.0 ml</td></tr>
<tr><td>Patient Name:</td><td></td><td>Age:</td><td></td></tr>
<tr><td>Sex:</td><td></td><td>Weight:</td><td></td></tr>
<tr><td colspan="4">Dose: As directed by the physician.</td></tr>
<tr><td>Mfg. Date:</td><td></td><td>Exp. Date:</td><td></td></tr>
<tr><td>Batch No.:</td><td></td><td>Price:</td><td></td></tr>
<tr><td colspan="4">Prepared by:

</td></tr>
</table>

Date :_____________   Marks : ________/10

EXPERIMENT NO. 65

- **Aim:** To prepare ________ ml codeine phosphate syrup.

- **Theory:** Syrups are concentrated oral solutions of sugar or nearly saturated solutions of sucrose in water. 65% w/w syrups retard the growth of microorganisms. It is important to note that sucrose concentration should not reach the saturation point, as a saturated solution may lead to crystallization of sucrose. Syrups are classified into the classes like simple syrups, medicated syrups, flavoured syrups.

  Codeine phosphate is the drug used as analgesic and anti-tussive. This preparation is generally used for the relief of cough and pain.

  Category: Analgesic and anti-tussive.

  Dose: 2 to 8 ml.

- **Procedure:** Dissolve weighed amount of codeine phosphate in purified water. Add chloroform spirit and mix thoroughly. Add 75 ml of syrup and mix it. Add sufficient amount of syrup to make 100 ml. Keep in a well-closed narrow-mouthed amber coloured bottle with suitable label.

- **Storage:** Preserve in a well-closed container.

VIVA VOCE QUESTIONS

Q.1   What is codeine phosphate?

____

Q.2   Give pharmaceutical applications of codeine phosphate.

____

Q.3   What is the dose of codeine phosphate syrup?

____

❖ ❖ ❖

Formulation Table:

Ingredients	Quantity required for 100 ml	Quantity required for _____ ml
Acacia	10.0 g	_____ g
Sodium benzoate	0.1 g	_____ g
Vanilla tincture	0.5 ml	_____ ml
Sucrose	80.0 g	_____ g
Water QS	100.0 ml	_____ ml

Calculations:

Acacia required to prepare 100 ml of syrup = 10 g

So, for preparation of _____ ml syrup, Acacia required $= \dfrac{10}{100} \times$ —— = —— g

Sodium benzoate required to prepare 100 ml of syrup = 0.1 g

So, for preparation of _____ ml syrup, Sodium benzoate required $= \dfrac{0.1}{100} \times$ —— = —— g

Vanilla tincture required to prepare 100 ml of syrup = 0.5 ml

So, for preparation of _____ ml syrup, Vanilla tincture required $= \dfrac{0.5}{100} \times$ —— = —— 0.1 ml

Label of Preparation:

CODEINE PHOSPHATE SYRUP			
Each 100 ml contains			
Acacia : 10.0 g Sodium benzoate : 0.1 g Vanilla tincture : 0.5 ml Sucrose : 80.0 g Water QS : 100.0 ml			
Patient Name:		**Age:**	
Sex:		**Weight:**	
Dose: As directed by the physician.			
Mfg. Date:		**Exp. Date:**	
Batch No.:		**Price:**	
Prepared by:			

Date :___________   Marks : ________/10

EXPERIMENT NO. 66

- **Aim:** To prepare _________ ml acacia syrup.
- **Theory:** Syrups are concentrated oral solutions of sugar or nearly saturated solutions of sucrose in water. 65% w/w syrups retard the growth of microorganisms. It is important to note that sucrose concentration should not reach the saturation point, as a saturated solution may lead to crystallization of sucrose. Syrups are classified into the classes like simple syrups, medicated syrups, flavoured syrups.

  Category: Pharmaceutical aid.

- **Procedure:** Mix the acacia powder, sodium benzoate and sucrose. Add 42.5 ml of purified water and mix thoroughly. Heat the mixture on steam bath until solubilized. Cool the solution and remove the scum. Mix vanilla tincture and sufficient amount of purified water to make 100 ml. Make homogeneous syrup and fill in suitable container.

- **Storage:** Preserve in a well-closed container.

VIVA VOCE QUESTIONS

Q.1   What is the use of acacia syrup?

____

Q.2   What is acacia?

____

Q.3   Why vanilla tincture is added in the syrup?

____

❖❖❖

Formulation Table:

Ingredients	Quantity required
Oleic acid	8.5 ml
Turpentine oil	25 ml
Dilute ammonia solution	4.5 ml
Ammonium chloride	1.25 g
Purified water	62.5 ml

Label of Preparation:

WHITE LINIMENT		
Each 100 ml contains		
Oleic acid : 8.5 ml		
Turpentine oil : 25 ml		
Dilute ammonia solution : 4.5 ml		
Ammonium chloride : 1.25 g		
Purified water : 62.5 ml		
Patient name:		**Age:**
Sex:		**Weight:**
Dose: As directed by the physician.		
Mfg. date:		**Exp. Date:**
Batch no.:		**Price:**
Prepared by:		

Date :______________   Marks :________/10

EXPERIMENT NO. 67

- **Aim:** To prepare white liniment.

- **Theory:** Liniments are solution or mixture of various substances in oil, alcoholic solutions of soap or emulsions or occasionally semi-solid preparations intended for external applications. They are applied with rubbing or massaged into skin as counter irritating or stimulating agents to the affected area. Some liniments are applied on a warm dressing or with a brush. The liniments may have uses like analgesic, antimicrobial, rubefacient, counter irritant, stimulants, and soothing agents. Two types of vehicles are used for preparation of liniments : alcohols and oils.

  Uses: Counter irritants.

  Dose: Directed by physician.

- **Procedure:** Mix oleic acid with measured quantity of turpentine oil. Mix dilute ammonia solution with 4.5 ml of purified water and warm it. Add warm diluted ammonia solution to the oily solution and shake to form an emulsion. Dissolve ammonium chloride in remaining amount of purified water. Mix this solution in the emulsion and shake it.

- **Storage:** Store in narrow mouthed coloured glass bottle.

VIVA VOCE QUESTIONS

Q.1   What is liniment?

____

Q.2   What are the uses of liniments?

____

Q.3   What is counter irritant?

____

❖ ❖ ❖

Formulation Table:

Ingredients	Quantity required
Camphor	20 g
Arachis oil	80 g

Label of Preparation:

CAMPHOR LINIMENT			
Each 100 g contains Camphor : 20 g Arachis oil : 80 g			
Patient name:		**Age:**	
Sex:		**Weight:**	
Dose: As directed by the physician.			
Mfg. date:		**Exp. Date:**	
Batch no.:		**Price:**	
Prepared by:			

Date :______________   Marks : __________/10

EXPERIMENT NO. 68

- **Aim:** To prepare camphor liniment.

- **Theory:** Camphor is a ketone, obtained from *cinnamomum camphora* Linn. It is in the form of colourless or white crystals, granules or crystalline masses. It is volatile in nature. So the preparation of camphor liniments should be stored out in a well-closed container at cool place. Arachis oil is obtained from the seed kennels of one or more of the cultivated varieties of *arachis hypogaea* Linn. It is used as a solvent for the preparations of various pharmaceutical products.

  Liniments are solution or mixture of various substances in oil, alcoholic solution of soap or emulsions or occasionally semi-solid preparations intended for external applications. They are applied with rubbing or massaged into skin as counter irritating or stimulating agents to the affected area. Some liniments are applied on a warm dressing or with a brush. The liniments may have uses like analgesic, antimicrobial, rubefacient, counter irritant, stimulants, and soothing agents. Two types of vehicles are used for preparation of liniments : alcohols and oils.

  Uses: Counter irritants.

- **Procedure:** Mix weighed amount of camphor in arachis oil in a closed vessel.

- **Storage:** Preserve in a well-closed glass container and store in cool place.

VIVA VOCE QUESTIONS

Q.1   What is the use of camphor liniment?

____

Q.2   Why liniments should be stored in a closed container?

____

Q.3   Why arachis oil is used in this liniment?

____

❖ ❖ ❖

Formulation Table:

Ingredients	Quantity required
Soft soap	8 g
Camphor	4 g
Lemon grass oil	1.5 g
Purified water	17 ml
Alcohol (90%) sufficient to produce	100 ml

Label of Preparation:

SOAP LINIMENT			
Each 100 ml contains			
Soft soap　　　　　　　　　　　　　　:　8 g			
Camphor　　　　　　　　　　　　　　:　4 g			
Lemon grass oil　　　　　　　　　　:　1.5 g			
Purified water　　　　　　　　　　　:　17 ml			
Alcohol (90%) sufficient to produce :　100 ml			
Patient name:		**Age:**	
Sex:		**Weight:**	
Dose: As directed by the physician.			
Mfg. date:		**Exp. Date:**	
Batch no.:		**Price:**	
Prepared by:			

Date :___________   Marks : _________/10

EXPERIMENT NO. 69

- **Aim:** To prepare soap liniment.

- **Theory:** Liniments are solution or mixture of various substances in oil, alcoholic solution of soap or emulsions or occasionally semi-solid preparations intended for external applications. They are applied with rubbing or massaged into skin as counter irritating or stimulating agents to the affected area. Some liniments are applied on a warm dressing or with a brush. The liniments may have uses like analgesic, antimicrobial, rubefacient, counter irritant, stimulants, and soothing agents. Two types of vehicles are used for preparation of liniments : alcohols and oils.

  Uses: Mild local irritants.

- **Procedure:** Dissolve the weighed quantity of soft soap, camphor and lemon grass oil in 60 ml of alcohol. Add purified water and remaining amount of alcohol to make up the volume and mix. Keep aside for a week and then filter to remove the undissolved substance.

- **Storage:** Preserve in a well-closed container.

VIVA VOCE QUESTIONS

Q.1   What is the use of soap liniment?

____

Q.2   How will you prepare soap liniment?

____

Q.3   What is the use of lemon grass oil?

____

❖ ❖ ❖

Formulation Table:

Ingredients	Quantity required
Soft soap	9 g
Camphor	5 g
Turpentine oil	65 ml
Purified water sufficient to produce	100 ml

Label of Preparation:

TURPENTINE LINIMENT		
Each 100 ml contains		
Soft soap	:	9 g
Camphor	:	5 g
Turpentine oil	:	65 ml
Purified water sufficient to produce	:	100 ml

Patient name:		Age:	
Sex:		Weight:	
Dose: As directed by the physician.			
Mfg. date:		Exp. Date:	
Batch no.:		Price:	
Prepared by:			

Date :__________   Marks : _________/10

EXPERIMENT NO. 70

- **Aim:** To prepare turpentine liniment.

- **Theory:** Turpentine oil is a colourless, limpid liquid with characteristic odour, pungent taste and somewhat bitter. On exposure to air, it undergoes oxidation reaction, which alters its colour and viscosity.

  Liniments are solution or mixture of various substances in oil, alcoholic solution of soap or emulsions or occasionally semi-solid preparations intended for external applications. They are applied with rubbing or massaged into skin as counter irritating or stimulating agents to the affected area. Some liniments are applied on a warm dressing or with a brush. The liniments may have uses like analgesic, antimicrobial, rubefacient, counter irritant, stimulants, and soothing agents. Two types of vehicles are used for preparation of liniments : alcohols and oils.

  Uses: Counter irritants and rubefacient.

- **Procedure:** Mix the soft soap with small amount of purified water (10 ml). Make solution of camphor in fresh rectified turpentine oil. Gradually add camphor solution to the soap mixture with trituration until a thick creamy emulsion is formed. Add sufficient amount of purified water to make up the volume and mix.

- **Storage:** Store in a well-closed container protected from light at a cool place.

VIVA VOCE QUESTIONS

Q.1   What is the use of turpentine liniment?

____

Q.2   How will you prepare turpentine liniment?

____

Q.3   What is counter irritant and rubefacient?

____

❖ ❖ ❖

Formulation Table:

Ingredients	Quantity required
Belladonna liquid extract	50 ml
Camphor	5 g
Alcohol (80%)	50 ml

Label of Preparation:

<table>
<tr><td colspan="4" align="center">BELLADONNA LINIMENT</td></tr>
<tr><td colspan="4">Each 100 ml contains
Belladonna liquid extract   :   50 ml
Camphor   :   5 g
Alcohol (80%)   :   50 ml</td></tr>
<tr><td>Patient name:</td><td></td><td>Age:</td><td></td></tr>
<tr><td>Sex:</td><td></td><td>Weight:</td><td></td></tr>
<tr><td colspan="4">Dose: As directed by the physician.</td></tr>
<tr><td>Mfg. date:</td><td></td><td>Exp. Date:</td><td></td></tr>
<tr><td>Batch no.:</td><td></td><td>Price:</td><td></td></tr>
<tr><td colspan="4">Prepared by:</td></tr>
</table>

Date :_____________   Marks : _________/10

EXPERIMENT NO. 71

- **Aim:** To prepare belladonna liniment.

- **Theory:** Liniments are solution or mixture of various substances in oil, alcoholic solution of soap or emulsions or occasionally semi-solid preparations intended for external applications. They are applied with rubbing or massaged into skin as counter irritating or stimulating agents to the affected area. Some liniments are applied on a warm dressing or with a brush. The liniments may have uses like analgesic, antimicrobial, rubefacient, counter irritant, stimulants, and soothing agents. Two types of vehicles are used for preparation of liniments : alcohols and oils.

  Uses: Local anaesthetic and parasympatholytic.

- **Procedure:** Dissolve belladonna liquid extract in alcohol. Add camphor in the mixture and mix it. Add remaining quantity of alcohol to make up the volume.

- **Storage:** Store in a well-closed container protected from light.

VIVA VOCE QUESTIONS

Q.1   What is the use of belladonna liniment?

____

Q.2   How will you prepare belladonna liniment?

____

Q.3   What is meaning of local anaesthetic?

____

❖❖❖

Formulation Table:

Ingredients	Quantity required
Calamine	5 g
Wool fat	1 g
Oleic acid	0.5 ml
Arachis oil	50 ml
Calcium hydroxide solution	100 ml

Label of Preparation:

CALAMINE LINIMENT			
Each 100 ml contains			
Calamine : 5 g			
Wool fat : 1 g			
Oleic acid : 0.5 ml			
Arachis oil : 50 ml			
Calcium hydroxide solution : 100 ml			
Patient name:		**Age:**	
Sex:		**Weight:**	
Dose: As directed by the physician.			
Mfg. date:		**Exp. Date:**	
Batch no.:		**Price:**	
Prepared by:			

Date :___________   Marks : _________/10

EXPERIMENT NO. 72

- **Aim:** To prepare calamine liniment.
- **Theory:** Liniments are solution or mixture of various substances in oil, alcoholic solution of soap or emulsions or occasionally semi-solid preparations intended for external applications. They are applied with rubbing or massaged into skin as counter irritating or stimulating agents to the affected area. Some liniments are applied on a warm dressing or with a brush. The liniments may have uses like analgesic, antimicrobial, rubefacient, counter irritant, stimulants, and soothing agents. Two types of vehicles are used for preparation of liniments : alcohols and oils.

  Uses: Rubefacient.
- **Procedure:** Melt weighed amount of wool fat, oleic acid and arachis oil. Triturate calamine with the melted oil. Add calcium hydroxide solution and shake it. Transfer it to a suitable container and shake vigorously.
- **Storage:** Store in a well-closed container protected from light.

VIVA VOCE QUESTIONS

Q.1   What is the use of calamine liniment?

____

Q.2   How will you prepare calamine liniment?

____

Q.3   What is the difference between lotion and liniment?

____

❖ ❖ ❖

Formulation Table:

Ingredients	Quantity required
Calamine	15 g
Zinc oxide	5 g
Bentonite	3 g
Sodium citrate	0.5 ml
Liquefied phenol	0.5 ml
Glycerin	5 ml
Rose water, sufficient to produce	100 ml

Label of Preparation:

<table>
<tr><td colspan="4" align="center">CALAMINE LOTION</td></tr>
<tr><td colspan="4">Each 100 ml contains</td></tr>
<tr><td colspan="4">Calamine   : 15 g</td></tr>
<tr><td colspan="4">Zinc oxide   : 5 g</td></tr>
<tr><td colspan="4">Bentonite   : 3 g</td></tr>
<tr><td colspan="4">Sodium citrate   : 0.5 ml</td></tr>
<tr><td colspan="4">Liquefied phenol   : 0.5 ml</td></tr>
<tr><td colspan="4">Glycerin   : 5 ml</td></tr>
<tr><td colspan="4">Rose water, sufficient to produce : 100 ml</td></tr>
<tr><td>Patient name:</td><td></td><td>Age:</td><td></td></tr>
<tr><td>Sex:</td><td></td><td>Weight:</td><td></td></tr>
<tr><td colspan="4">Dose: As directed by the physician.</td></tr>
<tr><td>Mfg. date:</td><td></td><td>Exp. Date:</td><td></td></tr>
<tr><td>Batch no.:</td><td></td><td>Price:</td><td></td></tr>
<tr><td colspan="4">Prepared by:</td></tr>
</table>

Date :____________   Marks : ________/10

EXPERIMENT NO. 73

- **Aim:** To prepare calamine lotion.

- **Theory:** Lotions are usually liquids or liquid suspensions or semi-solid preparations containing one or more medicaments, intended to be applied to the uniform skin without friction. They are either dabbed on skin or applied on a suitable dressing and covered with waterproof substance to reduce the evaporation. They may be prepared by triturating the ingredients to a smooth paste and then gradually adding the remaining liquid phase. Generally following substances are used in preparation of lotions : (i) Bentonite as suspending agent, (ii) Methyl cellulose or sodium carboxymethyl cellulose to hold the active ingredients in contact with the affected site, (iii) Glycerin as moistening agent, (iv) Alcohol as drying and cooling agent, (v) Rose water as vehicle and flavouring agent. Lotions may be used as anaesthetics, antiseptics, astringents, germicides, protective, antihistaminic and screening agents.

  Uses: Protective.

- **Procedure:** Prepare sodium citrate solution in 70 ml rose water. Triturate calamine, zinc oxide and bentonite with citrate solution. Add liquefied phenol and mix. Add glycerin and sufficient rose water to produce 100 ml.

- **Storage:** Store in a well-closed container.

VIVA VOCE QUESTIONS

Q.1   What is the use of calamine lotion?

____

Q.2   How will you prepare calamine lotion?

____

Q.3   How lotion is applied on skin?

____

❖ ❖ ❖

Formulation Table:

Ingredients	Quantity required
Chlorinated lime	1.25 g
Boric acid	1.25 g
Purified water, sufficient to produce	100 ml

Label of Preparation:

BORIC ACID LOTION			
Each 100 ml contains			
Chlorinated lime : 1.25 g			
Boric acid : 1.25 g			
Purified water, sufficient to produce : 100 ml			
Patient name:		**Age:**	
Sex:		**Weight:**	
Dose: As directed by the physician.			
Mfg. date:		**Exp. Date:**	
Batch no.:		**Price:**	
Prepared by:			

Date :___________   Marks : ________/10

EXPERIMENT NO. 74

- **Aim:** To prepare boric acid lotion.

- **Theory:** Lotions are usually liquids or liquid suspensions or semi-solid preparations containing one or more medicaments, intended to be applied to the uniform skin without friction. They are either dabbed on skin or applied on a suitable dressing and covered with waterproof substance to reduce the evaporation. They may be prepared by triturating the ingredients to a smooth paste and then gradually adding the remaining liquid phase. Generally following substances are used in preparation of lotions : (i) Bentonite as suspending agent, (ii) Methyl cellulose or sodium carboxymethyl cellulose to hold the active ingredients in contact with the affected site, (iii) Glycerin as moistening agent, (iv) Alcohol as drying and cooling agent, (v) Rose water as vehicle and flavouring agent. Lotions may be used as anaesthetics, antiseptics, astringents, germicides, protective, antihistaminic and screening agents.

    Uses: Local anti-infective, germicide.

- **Procedure:** Mix chlorinated lime and boric acid. Dissolve in purified water and add sufficient water to produce 100 ml.

- **Storage:** Store in a well-closed container.

VIVA VOCE QUESTIONS

Q.1   What is the use of Boric acid lotion?

____

Q.2   How will you prepare boric acid lotion?

____

Q.3   What is the difference between lotion and liniments?

____

❖ ❖ ❖

Formulation Table:

Ingredients	Quantity required
Cetrimide	1 mg
Purified water, sufficient to produce	100 ml

Label of Preparation:

<table>
<tr><td colspan="4" align="center">CETRIMIDE LOTION</td></tr>
<tr><td colspan="4">Each 100 ml contains
Cetrimide   :   1 mg
Purified water, sufficient to produce   :   100 ml</td></tr>
<tr><td>Patient name:</td><td></td><td>Age:</td><td></td></tr>
<tr><td>Sex:</td><td></td><td>Weight:</td><td></td></tr>
<tr><td colspan="4">Dose: As directed by the physician.</td></tr>
<tr><td>Mfg. date:</td><td></td><td>Exp. Date:</td><td></td></tr>
<tr><td>Batch no.:</td><td></td><td>Price:</td><td></td></tr>
<tr><td colspan="4">Prepared by:</td></tr>
</table>

Date :___________   Marks : ________/10

EXPERIMENT NO. 75

- **Aim:** To prepare cetrimide lotion.

- **Theory:** Lotions are usually liquids or liquid suspensions or semi-solid preparations containing one or more medicaments, intended to be applied to the uniform skin without friction. They are either dabbed on skin or applied on a suitable dressing and covered with waterproof substance to reduce the evaporation. They may be prepared by triturating the ingredients to a smooth paste and then gradually adding the remaining liquid phase. Generally following substances are used in preparation of lotions : (i) Bentonite as suspending agent, (ii) Methyl cellulose or sodium carboxymethyl cellulose to hold the active ingredients in contact with the affected site, (iii) Glycerin as moistening agent, (iv) Alcohol as drying and cooling agent, (v) Rose water as vehicle and flavouring agent. Lotions may be used as anaesthetics, antiseptics, astringents, germicides, protective, antihistaminic and screening agents.

  Uses: Anti-bacterial.

- **Procedure:** Dissolve cetrimide in purified water and make up the volume using purified water.

- **Storage:** Store in a well-closed container.

VIVA VOCE QUESTIONS

Q.1   What is the use of cetrimide lotion?

____

Q.2   How will you prepare cetrimide lotion?

____

Q.3   What is the meaning of anti-bacterial?

____

❖ ❖ ❖

Formulation Table:

Ingredients	Quantity required
Zinc sulphate	1 g
Amaranth solution	1 ml
Purified water, sufficient to produce	100 ml

Label of Preparation:

ZINC SULPHATE LOTION			
Each 100 ml contains			
Zinc sulphate : 1 g			
Amaranth solution : 1 ml			
Purified water, sufficient to produce : 100 ml			
Patient name:		**Age:**	
Sex:		**Weight:**	
Dose: As directed by the physician.			
Mfg. date:		**Exp. Date:**	
Batch no.:		**Price:**	
Prepared by:			

Date :___________   Marks : ________/10

EXPERIMENT NO. 76

- **Aim:** To prepare zinc sulphate lotion.

- **Theory:** Lotions are usually liquids or liquid suspensions or semi-solid preparations containing one or more medicaments, intended to be applied to the uniform skin without friction. They are either dabbed on skin or applied on a suitable dressing and covered with waterproof substance to reduce the evaporation. They may be prepared by triturating the ingredients to a smooth paste and then gradually adding the remaining liquid phase. Generally following substances are used in preparation of lotions : (i) Bentonite as suspending agent, (ii) Methyl cellulose or sodium carboxymethyl cellulose to hold the active ingredients in contact with the affected site, (iii) Glycerin as moistening agent, (iv) Alcohol as drying and cooling agent, (v) Rose water as vehicle and flavouring agent. Lotions may be used as anaesthetics, antiseptics, astringents, germicides, protective, antihistaminic and screening agents.

  Uses: Protective.

- **Procedure:** Dissolve zinc sulphate in purified water. Add amaranth solution and mix. Make up the volume using purified water.

- **Storage:** Store in a well-closed container.

VIVA VOCE QUESTIONS

Q.1   What is the use of zinc sulphate lotion?

____

Q.2   How will you prepare zinc sulphate lotion?

____

Q.3   What is the meaning of protective?

____

❖❖❖

Formulation Table:

Ingredients	Quantity required
Potassium permanganate	1 g
Purified water, sufficient to produce	100 ml

Label of Preparation:

POTASSIUM PERMANGANATE LOTION			
Each 100 ml contains			
Potassium permanganate : 1 g Purified water, sufficient to produce : 100 ml			
Patient name:		**Age:**	
Sex:		**Weight:**	
Dose: As directed by the physician.			
Mfg. date:		**Exp. Date:**	
Batch no.:		**Price:**	
Prepared by:			

Date :_____________   Marks : _________/10

EXPERIMENT NO. 77

- **Aim:** To prepare potassium permanganate lotion.

- **Theory:** Lotions are usually liquids or liquid suspensions or semi-solid preparations containing one or more medicaments, intended to be applied to the uniform skin without friction. They are either dabbed on skin or applied on a suitable dressing and covered with waterproof substance to reduce the evaporation. They may be prepared by triturating the ingredients to a smooth paste and then gradually adding the remaining liquid phase. Generally following substances are used in preparation of lotions : (1) Bentonite as suspending agent, (ii) Methyl cellulose or sodium carboxymethyl cellulose to hold the active ingredients in contact with the affected site (iii) Glycerin as moistening agent, (iv) Alcohol as drying and cooling agent, (v) Rose water as vehicle and flavouring agent. Lotions may be used as anaesthetics, antiseptics, astringents, germicides, protective, antihistaminic and screening agents.

  Uses: Anti-septic.

- **Procedure:** Triturate potassium permanganate with purified water. Add sufficient purified water to produce 100 ml.

- **Storage:** Store in a well-closed container. Must be freshly prepared. Dilute with 7 parts of water as directed.

VIVA VOCE QUESTIONS

Q.1   What is the use of potassium permanganate lotion?

____

Q.2   How will you prepare potassium permanganate lotion?

____

Q.3   What is meaning of anti-septic ?

____

❖❖❖

Formulation Table:

Ingredients	Quantity required
Calamine, finely powdered	1.5 g
White soft paraffin	8.5 g

Label of Preparation:

CALAMINE OINTMENT			
Each 10 g contains Calamine : 1.5 g White soft paraffin : 8.5 g			
Patient name:		**Age:**	
Sex:		**Weight:**	
Dose: As directed by the physician.			
Mfg. date:		**Exp. Date:**	
Batch no.:		**Price:**	
Prepared by:			

Date :___________   Marks : _________/10

EXPERIMENT NO. 78

- **Aim:** To prepare calamine ointment.

- **Theory:** Ointments are semi-solid preparations for application to the skin. They are often anhydrous and contain the medicament either dissolved or dispersed in the vehicle. The solid substances, which are dispersed, should be in the form of a microionized powder. They are easily spread and their plastic viscosity may be controlled by modifications of the formulations.

  Uses: Astringent and protective.

- **Procedure:** Triturate the calamine powder with part of the white soft paraffin until smooth. Add gradually sufficient quantity of white soft paraffin to produce 10 g.

- **Storage:** Preserve in a well-closed container.

VIVA VOCE QUESTIONS

Q.1   What is the use of calamine ointment?

____

Q.2   Why ointments are required?

____

❖ ❖ ❖

Formulation Table:

Ingredients	Quantity required for 100 g	Quantity required for ______ g
White bees wax	2.0 g	______ g
Hard paraffin	3.0 g	______ g
Cetostearyl alcohol	5.0 g	______ g
White soft paraffin	90.0 g	______ g

Calculations:

White bees wax required to prepare 100 g of ointment = 2.0 g

So, for preparation of ______ ml ointment, white bees wax required = $\dfrac{2}{100} \times \underline{\quad} = \underline{\quad}$ g

Hard paraffin required to prepare 100 g of ointment = 3.0 g

So, for preparation of ______ ml ointment, Hard paraffin required = $\dfrac{3}{100} \times \underline{\quad} = \underline{\quad}$ g

Cetostearyl alcohol required to prepare 100 g of ointment = 5.0 g

So, for preparation of ______ ml ointment, Cetostearyl alcohol required = $\dfrac{5}{100} \times \underline{\quad} = \underline{\quad}$ g

White soft paraffin required to prepare 100 g of ointment = 90.0 g

So, for preparation of ______ ml ointment, White soft paraffin required = $\dfrac{90}{100} \times \underline{\quad} = \underline{\quad}$ g

Label of Preparation:

EMULSIFYING OINTMENT			
Each 100 g contains			
White bees wax : 2.0 g Hard paraffin : 3.0 g Cetostearyl alcohol : 5.0 g White soft paraffin : 90.0 g			
Patient Name:		**Age:**	
Sex:		**Weight:**	
Dose: As directed by the physician.			
Mfg. Date:		**Exp. Date:**	
Batch No.:		**Price:**	
Prepared by:			

Date :___________   Marks : ________/10

EXPERIMENT NO. 79

- **Aim:** To prepare _______ g emulsifying ointment.

- **Theory:** Ointments are semi-solid preparations for application to the skin. They are often anhydrous and contain the medicament either dissolved or dispersed in the vehicle. The solid substances, which are dispersed, should be in the form of a microionized powder. They are easily spread and their plastic viscosity may be controlled by modifications of the formulations.

  Uses: Pharmaceutical aid.

- **Procedure:** Melt the white bees wax on water bath. Mix the hard paraffin, cetostearyl alcohol and white soft paraffin. Stir them all until cool. After cooling transfer the ointment in suitable container.

- **Storage:** Preserve in a well-closed container, and protect from light.

VIVA VOCE QUESTIONS

Q.1   What is the use of emulsifying ointment?

____

Q.2   What is difference between cream and ointment?

____

❖ ❖ ❖

Formulation Table:

Ingredients	Quantity required for 100 g	Quantity required for _____ g
Cetrimide	3.0 g	_____ g
White soft paraffin	50.0 g	_____ g
Cetostearyl alcohol	27.0 g	_____ g
Liquid paraffin	20.0 g	_____ g

Calculations:

Cetrimide required to prepare 100 g of ointment = 3.0 g

So, for preparation of ____ g ointment, Cetrimide required = $\dfrac{3}{100} \times$ —— = —— g

White soft paraffin required to prepare 100 g of ointment = 50.0 g

So, for preparation of ____ g ointment, White soft paraffin required = $\dfrac{50}{100} \times$ —— = —— g

Cetostearyl alcohol required to prepare 100 g of ointment = 27.0 g

So, for preparation of ____ g ointment, Cetostearyl alcohol required = $\dfrac{27}{100} \times$ —— = —— g

Liquid paraffin required to prepare 100 g of ointment = 20.0 g

So, for preparation of ____ g ointment, Liquid paraffin required = $\dfrac{20}{100} \times$ —— = —— g

Label of Preparation:

<table>
<tr><td colspan="4" align="center">CETRIMIDE EMULSIFYING OINTMENT</td></tr>
<tr><td colspan="4">Each 100 g contains</td></tr>
<tr><td colspan="4">Cetrimide   : 3.0 g
White soft paraffin   : 50.0 g
Cetostearyl alcohol : 27.0 g
Liquid paraffin   : 20.0 g</td></tr>
<tr><td>Patient Name:</td><td></td><td>Age:</td><td></td></tr>
<tr><td>Sex:</td><td></td><td>Weight:</td><td></td></tr>
<tr><td colspan="4">Dose: As directed by the physician.</td></tr>
<tr><td>Mfg. Date:</td><td></td><td>Exp. Date:</td><td></td></tr>
<tr><td>Batch No.:</td><td></td><td>Price:</td><td></td></tr>
<tr><td colspan="4">Prepared by:</td></tr>
</table>

Date :___________   Marks : ________/10

EXPERIMENT NO. 80

- **Aim:** To prepare _______ g cetrimide emulsifying ointment.

- **Theory:** Ointments are semi-solid preparations for application to the skin. They are often anhydrous and contain the medicament either dissolved or dispersed in the vehicle. The solid substances, which are dispersed, should be in the form of a microionized powder. They are easily spread and their plastic viscosity may be controlled by modifications of the formulations.

  Uses: Protective.

- **Procedure:** Melt together white soft paraffin, cetostearyl alcohol, and liquid paraffin. Add powdered cetrimide in base and stir until cold.

- **Storage:** Preserve in a well-closed container and store in cool place.

VIVA VOCE QUESTIONS

Q.1   What is the use of cetrimide emulsifying ointment?

____

Q.2   What is the difference between gel and ointment?

____

❖ ❖ ❖

Formulation Table:

Ingredients	Quantity required for 100 g	Quantity required for _____ g
Wool fat	5.0 g	_____ g
Cetostearyl alcohol	5.0 g	_____ g
Hard Paraffin	5.0 g	_____ g
White soft paraffin	85.0 g	_____ g

Calculations:

Wool fat required to prepare 100 g of ointment = 5.0 g

So, for preparation of _____ g ointment, Wool fat required = $\dfrac{5}{100} \times \dfrac{\quad}{\quad} = \dfrac{\quad}{\quad}$ g

Cetostearyl alcohol required to prepare 100 g of ointment = 5.0 g

So, for preparation of _____ g ointment, Cetostearyl alcohol required = $\dfrac{5}{100} \times \dfrac{\quad}{\quad} = \dfrac{\quad}{\quad}$ g

Hard Paraffin required to prepare 100 g of ointment = 5.0 g

So, for preparation of _____ g ointment, Hard Paraffin required = $\dfrac{5}{100} \times \dfrac{\quad}{\quad} = \dfrac{\quad}{\quad}$ g

White soft paraffin required to prepare 100 g of ointment = 85.0 g

So, for preparation of _____ g ointment, White soft paraffin required = $\dfrac{85}{100} \times \dfrac{\quad}{\quad} = \dfrac{\quad}{\quad}$ g

Label of Preparation:

SIMPLE OINTMENT		
Each 100 g contains		
Wool fat : 5.0 g		
Cetostearyl alcohol : 5.0 g		
Hard paraffin : 5.0 g		
White soft paraffin : 85.0 g		
Patient Name:		**Age:**
Sex:		**Weight:**
Dose: As directed by the physician.		
Mfg. Date:		**Exp. Date:**
Batch No.:		**Price:**
Prepared by:		

Date :___________   Marks : _________/10

EXPERIMENT NO. 81

- **Aim:** To prepare _______ g simple ointment.

- **Theory:** Ointments are semi-solid preparations for application to the skin. They are often anhydrous and contain the medicament either dissolved or dispersed in the vehicle. The solid substances, which are dispersed, should be in the form of a microionized powder. They are easily spread and their plastic viscosity may be controlled by modifications of the formulations.

  Uses: Pharmaceutical aid.

- **Procedure:** Mix wool fat, cetostearyl alcohol, hard paraffin, and white soft paraffin or yellow soft paraffin in a container. Heat the mixture gently with stirring until homogeneous. Stir continually until cold.

- **Storage:** Preserve in a well-closed container and store in cool place.

VIVA VOCE QUESTIONS

Q.1   What is the use of simple ointment?

____

Q.2   What is the difference between paste and ointment?

____

❖❖❖

Formulation Table:

Ingredients	Quantity required for 100 g	Quantity required for _____ g
White bees wax	10.0 g	_____ g
Hard paraffin	15.0 g	_____ g
Cetostearyl alcohol	25.0 g	_____ g
White soft paraffin	50.0 g	_____ g

Calculations:

White bees wax required to prepare 100 g of ointment = 10.0 g

So, for preparation of _____ g ointment, White bees wax required $= \dfrac{10}{100} \times$ —— = —— g

Hard paraffin required to prepare 100 g of ointment = 15.0 g

So, for preparation of _____ g ointment, Hard paraffin required $= \dfrac{15}{100} \times$ —— = —— g

Cetostearyl alcohol required to prepare 100 g of ointment = 25.0 g

So, for preparation of _____ g ointment, Cetostearyl alcohol required $= \dfrac{25}{100} \times$ — = — g

White soft paraffin required to prepare 100 g of ointment = 50.0 g

So, for preparation of _____ g ointment, White soft paraffin required $= \dfrac{50}{100} \times$ — = — g

Label of Preparation:

PARAFFIN OINTMENT			
Each 100 g contains			
White bees wax : 10.0 g Hard Paraffin : 15.0 g Cetostearyl alcohol : 25.0 g White soft paraffin : 50.0 g			
Patient Name:		**Age:**	
Sex:		**Weight:**	
Dose: As directed by the physician.			
Mfg. Date:		**Exp. Date:**	
Batch No.:		**Price:**	
Prepared by:			

Date :___________　　　　　　　　　　　　　　　　　　Marks : ________/10

EXPERIMENT NO. 82

- **Aim:** To prepare ________ g paraffin ointment.

- **Theory:** Ointments are semi-solid preparations for application to the skin. They are often anhydrous and contain the medicament either dissolved or dispersed in the vehicle. The solid substances, which are dispersed, should be in the form of a microionized powder. They are easily spread and their plastic viscosity may be controlled by modifications of the formulations.

  Uses: Pharmaceutical aid and protective.

- **Procedure:** Mix white bees wax, hard paraffin, cetostearyl alcohol, and white soft paraffin. Heat gently with stirring until homogeneous and stir until cold.

- **Storage:** Preserve in a well-closed container and store in cool place.

VIVA VOCE QUESTIONS

Q.1　　How do you prepare paraffin ointment?

____

Q.2　　What is the use of paraffin ointment?

____

❖ ❖ ❖

Formulation Table:

Ingredients	Quantity required for 100 g	Quantity required for _____ g
Precipitated sulphur	10.0 g	_____ g
Simple ointment	90.0 g	_____ g

Calculations:

Precipitated sulphur required to prepare 100 g of sulphur ointment = 10.0 g

So, for preparation of _____ g sulphur ointment, Precipitated sulphur required

$$= \frac{10}{100} \times \underline{\quad} = \underline{\quad} g$$

Simple ointment required to prepare 100 g of sulphur ointment = 90.0 g

So, for preparation of _____ g sulphur ointment, Simple ointment required

$$= \frac{90}{100} \times \underline{\quad} = \underline{\quad} g$$

Label of Preparation:

SULPHUR OINTMENT			
Each 100 g contains			
Precipitated sulphur	: 10.0 g		
Simple ointment	: 90.0 g		
Patient Name:		**Age:**	
Sex:		**Weight:**	
Dose: As directed by the physician.			
Mfg. Date:		**Exp. Date:**	
Batch No.:		**Price:**	
Prepared by:			

Date :___________   Marks :________/10

EXPERIMENT NO. 83

- **Aim:** To prepare _______ g sulphur ointment.

- **Theory:** Ointments are semi-solid preparations for application to the skin. They are often anhydrous and contain the medicament either dissolved or dispersed in the vehicle. The solid substances, which are dispersed, should be in the form of a microionized powder. They are easily spread and their plastic viscosity may be controlled by modifications of the formulations.

  Uses: Scabicide.

- **Procedure:** Triturate the precipitated sulphur with a portion of the simple ointment until smooth. Add gradually the remainder of the simple ointment and mix thoroughly.

- **Storage:** Preserve in a well-closed container and store in cool place.

VIVA VOCE QUESTIONS

Q.1   How do you prepare sulphur ointment?

____

Q.2   What is scabicide?

____

❖ ❖ ❖

Formulation Table:

Ingredients	Quantity required for 100 g	Quantity required for _____ g
Zinc oxide	15.0 g	_____ g
Simple ointment	85.0 g	_____ g

Calculations:

Zinc oxide required to prepare 100 g of zinc ointment = 15.0 g

So, for preparation of _____ g zinc ointment, Zinc oxide required = $\dfrac{15}{100}$ × ——— = ——— g

Simple ointment required to prepare 100 g of zinc ointment = 85.0 g

So, for preparation of _____ g zinc ointment, Simple ointment required

$$= \dfrac{85}{100} × ——— = ——— \text{ g}$$

Label of Preparation:

<table>
<tr><td colspan="4" align="center">SULPHUR OINTMENT</td></tr>
<tr><td colspan="4">Each 100 g contains</td></tr>
<tr><td colspan="4">Zinc oxide   : 15.0 g</td></tr>
<tr><td colspan="4">Simple ointment   : 85.0 g</td></tr>
<tr><td>Patient Name:</td><td></td><td>Age:</td><td></td></tr>
<tr><td>Sex:</td><td></td><td>Weight:</td><td></td></tr>
<tr><td colspan="4">Dose: As directed by the physician.</td></tr>
<tr><td>Mfg. Date:</td><td></td><td>Exp. Date:</td><td></td></tr>
<tr><td>Batch No.:</td><td></td><td>Price:</td><td></td></tr>
<tr><td colspan="4">Prepared by:</td></tr>
</table>

Date :___________   Marks : _________/10

EXPERIMENT NO. 84

- **Aim:** To prepare ________ g zinc ointment.

- **Theory:** Ointments are semi-solid preparations for application to the skin. They are often anhydrous and contain the medicament either dissolved or dispersed in the vehicle. The solid substances, which are dispersed, should be in the form of a microionized powder. They are easily spread and their plastic viscosity may be controlled by modifications of the formulations.

  Uses: Astringent, protective and antiseptic.

- **Procedure:** Triturate the zinc oxide with a portion of the simple ointment until smooth. Gradually add simple ointment sufficient to produce desired amount.

- **Storage:** Preserve in a well-closed container and store in cool place.

VIVA VOCE QUESTIONS

Q.1   How do you prepare sulphur ointment?

____

Q.2   What is astringent?

____

❖ ❖ ❖

Formulation Table:

Ingredients	Quantity required for 10 ml	Quantity required for _____ mg
Methyl hydroxybenzoate	22.0 mg	_______ mg
Propyl hydroxybenzoate	11.4 mg	_______ mg
Purified water	10.0 ml	_______ ml

Calculations:

Methyl hydroxybenzoate required to prepare 10 ml of eye drops = 22.0 mg

So, for preparation of _______ ml eye drops, Methyl hydroxybenzoate required

$$= \frac{22}{10} \times \text{---} = \text{---} \text{ mg}$$

Propyl hydroxybenzoate required to prepare 10 ml of eye drops = 11.4 mg

So, for preparation of _______ ml eye drop, Propyl hydroxybenzoate required

$$= \frac{11.4}{10} \times \text{---} = \text{---} \text{ mg}$$

Label of Preparation:

SOLUTION FOR EYE DROPS			
Each 10 ml contains			
Methyl hydroxybenzoate : 22.0 mg			
Propyl hydroxybenzoate : 11.4 mg			
Purified water : 10.0 ml			
Patient Name:		**Age:**	
Sex:		**Weight:**	
Dose: As directed by the physician.			
Mfg. Date:		**Exp. Date:**	
Batch No.:		**Price:**	
Prepared by:			

Date :___________   Marks : ________/10

EXPERIMENT NO. 85

- **Aim:** To prepare _______ ml solution for eye drops.

- **Theory:** Eye drops must be freshly prepared aseptically and dispensed in previously sterilized container. A suitable fungistatic should be used in preparations liable to support the growth of moulds. For oily eye drops, the oily vehicle which has been previously sterilized by heating at 160°C for one hour must be used. Eye drops should be made approximately isotonic with lachrymal secretions by the addition of sodium chloride or other suitable substance. Care should be taken to avoid contamination during use.

  Uses: Pharmaceutical aid.

  Dose: As directed by physician.

- **Procedure:** Dissolve methyl hydroxybenzoate and propyl hydroxybenzoate in boiling water under aseptic conditions. Add freshly boiled and cooled purified water to produce the required volume.

- **Storage:** Preserve in a well-closed container and protect from light and contamination.

VIVA VOCE QUESTIONS

Q.1   How do you prepare eye drops?

____

Q.2   What is the difference between eye drops and eye lotion?

____

❖ ❖ ❖

Formulation Table:

Ingredients	Quantity required for 10 ml	Quantity required for _____ mg
Amethocaine hydrochloride	100.0 mg	______mg
Sodium chloride	68.0 mg	______ mg
Solution of eye drops	10.0 ml	_____ ml

Calculations:

Amethocaine hydrochloride required to prepare 10 ml of eye drops = 100.0 mg

So, for preparation of ______ ml eye drops, Amethocaine hydrochloride required

$$= \frac{100}{10} \times \text{——} = \text{——} \ mg$$

Sodium chloride required to prepare 10 ml of eye drops = 68.0 mg

So, for preparation of ______ ml eye drops, Sodium chloride required

$$= \frac{68}{10} \times \text{——} = \text{——} \ mg$$

Label of Preparation:

AMETHOCAINE FOR EYE DROP			
Each 10 ml contains			
Amethocaine hydrochloride : 100.0 mg			
Sodium chloride : 68.0 mg			
Solution of eye drops : 10.0 ml			
Patient Name:		**Age:**	
Sex:		**Weight:**	
Dose: As directed by the physician.			
Mfg. Date:		**Exp. Date:**	
Batch No.:		**Price:**	
Prepared by:			

Date : ___________   Marks : _________/10

EXPERIMENT NO. 86

- **Aim:** To prepare _______ ml amethocaine eye drops.

- **Theory:** Eye drops must be freshly prepared aseptically and dispensed in previously sterilized container. A suitable fungistatic should be used in preparations liable to support the growth of moulds. For oily eye drops, the oily vehicle which has been previously sterilized by heating at 160°C for one hour must be used. Eye drops should be made approximately isotonic with lachrymal secretions by the addition of sodium chloride or other suitable substance. Care should be taken to avoid contamination during use.

  Uses: Local anaesthetic.

  Dose: As directed by physician.

- **Procedure:** Dissolve sodium chloride in solution of eye drops and prepare a solution. Add amethocaine hydrochloride and dissolve it by shaking. Sterile by autoclave.

- **Storage:** Preserve in a well-closed container.

VIVA VOCE QUESTIONS

Q.1   What is local anaesthetic eye drops?

____

Q.2   How the preparation can be sterilized?

____

❖ ❖ ❖

Formulation Table:

Ingredients	Quantity required for 10 ml	Quantity required for _____ mg
Atropine sulphate	100.0 mg	_____mg
Sodium chloride	75.0 mg	_____ mg
Solution of eye drops	10.0 ml	_____ ml

Calculations:

Atropine sulphate required to prepare 10 ml of eye drops = 100.0 mg

So, for preparation of _______ ml eye drops, Atropine sulphate required

$$= \frac{100}{10} \times \text{------} = \text{------} \ mg$$

Sodium chloride required to prepare 10 ml of eye drops = 75.0 mg

So, for preparation of _______ ml eye drops, Sodium chloride required

$$= \frac{75}{10} \times \text{------} = \text{------} \ mg$$

Label of Preparation:

ATROPINE SULPHATE EYE DROP		
Each 10 ml contains		
Atropine sulphate : 100.0 mg		
Sodium chloride : 75.0 mg		
Solution of eye drop : 10.0 ml		
Patient Name:	**Age:**	
Sex:	**Weight:**	
Dose: As directed by the physician.		
Mfg. Date:	**Exp. Date:**	
Batch No.:	**Price:**	
Prepared by:		

Date :___________   Marks : _________/10

EXPERIMENT NO. 87

- **Aim:** To prepare _______ ml atropine eye drops.

- **Theory:** Eye drops must be freshly prepared aseptically and dispensed in previously sterilized container. A suitable fungistatic should be used in preparations liable to support the growth of moulds. For oily eye drops, the oily vehicle which has been previously sterilized by heating at 160°C for one hour must be used. Eye drops should be made approximately isotonic with lachrymal secretions by the addition of sodium chloride or other suitable substance. Care should be taken to avoid contamination during use.

  Uses: Antimuscarinic.

  Dose: As directed by physician.

- **Procedure:** Dissolve sodium chloride in solution of eye drops and prepare a solution. Add atropine sulphate and dissolve it by shaking. Sterile by autoclave.

- **Storage:** Preserve in a well-closed container.

VIVA VOCE QUESTIONS

Q.1   What is the use of atropine sulphate?

____

Q.2   Give storage condition of eye drops?

____

❖ ❖ ❖

Formulation Table:

Ingredients	Quantity required for 10 ml	Quantity required for _____mg
Cocaine hydrochloride	200.0 mg	_______mg
Sodium chloride	60.0 mg	_______ mg
Solution of eye drops	10.0 ml	_______ ml

Calculations:

Cocaine hydrochloride required to prepare 10 ml of eye drops =   200.0 mg

So, for preparation of _______ ml eye drops, Cocaine hydrochloride required

$$= \frac{200}{10} \times \text{------} = \text{------ mg}$$

Sodium chloride required to prepare 10 ml of eye drops =   60.0 mg

So, for preparation of _______ ml eye drops, Sodium chloride required

$$= \frac{60}{10} \times \text{------} = \text{------ mg}$$

Label of Preparation:

COCAINE HYDROCHLORIDE EYE DROP			
Each 10 ml contains			
Cocaine hydrochloride : 200.0 mg			
Sodium chloride : 60.0 mg			
Solution of eye drops : 10.0 ml			
Patient Name:		**Age:**	
Sex:		**Weight:**	
Dose: As directed by the physician.			
Mfg. Date:		**Exp. Date:**	
Batch No.:		**Price:**	
Prepared by:			

Date :__________ Marks : _________/10

EXPERIMENT NO. 88

- **Aim:** To prepare _______ ml cocaine hydrochloride eye drops.

- **Theory:** Eye drops must be freshly prepared aseptically and dispensed in previously sterilized container. A suitable fungistatic should be used in preparations liable to support the growth of moulds. For oily eye drops, the oily vehicle which has been previously sterilized by heating at 160ºC for one hour must be used. Eye drops should be made approximately isotonic with lachrymal secretions by the addition of sodium chloride or other suitable substance. Care should be taken to avoid contamination during use.

  Uses: Local anaesthetic.

  Dose: As directed by physician.

- **Procedure:** Dissolve sodium chloride in solution of eye drops and prepare a solution. Add cocaine hydrochloride and dissolve it by shaking. Sterile by autoclave.

- **Storage:** Preserve in a well-closed container.

VIVA VOCE QUESTIONS

Q.1   What is cocaine?

____

Q.2   What is local anaesthetic?

____

❖ ❖ ❖

Formulation Table:

Ingredients	Quantity required for 10 ml	Quantity required for _____ mg
Framycetin sulphate	50.0 mg	_______ mg
Sodium chloride	75.0 mg	_______ mg
Solution of eye drops	10.0 ml	_____ ml

Calculations:

Framycetin sulphate required to prepare 10 ml of eye drops = 50.0 mg

So, for preparation of _______ ml eye drops, Framycetin sulphate required

$$= \frac{50}{10} \times \text{\textemdash} = \text{\textemdash} \text{ mg}$$

Sodium chloride required to prepare 10 ml of eye drops = 75.0 mg

So, for preparation of _______ ml eye drops, Sodium chloride required

$$= \frac{75}{10} \times \text{\textemdash} = \text{\textemdash} \text{ mg}$$

Label of Preparation:

<table>
<tr><td colspan="4" align="center">FRAMYCETIN SULPHATE EYE DROPS</td></tr>
<tr><td colspan="4">Each 10 ml contains</td></tr>
<tr><td colspan="4">Framycetin sulphate   : 50.0 mg</td></tr>
<tr><td colspan="4">Sodium chloride   : 75.0 mg</td></tr>
<tr><td colspan="4">Solution of eye drops   : 10.0 ml</td></tr>
<tr><td>Patient Name:</td><td></td><td>Age:</td><td></td></tr>
<tr><td>Sex:</td><td></td><td>Weight:</td><td></td></tr>
<tr><td colspan="4">Dose: As directed by the physician.</td></tr>
<tr><td>Mfg. Date:</td><td></td><td>Exp. Date:</td><td></td></tr>
<tr><td>Batch No.:</td><td></td><td>Price:</td><td></td></tr>
<tr><td colspan="4">Prepared by:</td></tr>
</table>

Date :___________   Marks : _________/10

EXPERIMENT NO. 89

- **Aim:** To prepare _______ ml framycetin eye drops.

- **Theory:** Eye drops must be freshly prepared aseptically and dispensed in previously sterilized container. A suitable fungistatic should be used in preparations liable to support the growth of moulds. For oily eye drops, the oily vehicle which has been previously sterilized by heating at 160ºC for one hour must be used. Eye drops should be made approximately isotonic with lachrymal secretions by the addition of sodium chloride or other suitable substance. Care should be taken to avoid contamination during use.

  Uses: Anti-microbial.

  Dose: As directed by physician.

- **Procedure:** Dissolve sodium chloride in solution of eye drops and prepare a solution. Add framycetin sulphate and dissolve it by shaking. Sterile by autoclave.

- **Storage:** Preserve in a well-closed container.

VIVA VOCE QUESTIONS

Q.1   What is eye drops?

____

Q.2   Which type of dosage form is more suitable for eye?

____

❖ ❖ ❖

Formulation Table:

Ingredients	Quantity required for 10 ml	Quantity required for _____ mg
Pilocarpine nitrate	100.0 mg	______mg
Sodium chloride	68.0 mg	______ mg
Solution of eye drops	10.0 ml	______ ml

Calculations:

Pilocarpine nitrate required to prepare 10 ml of eye drops = 100.0 mg

So, for preparation of _______ ml eye drops, Pilocarpine nitrate required

$$= \frac{100}{10} \times \text{———} = \text{———} \text{ mg}$$

Sodium chloride required to prepare 10 ml of eye drops = 68.0 mg

So, for preparation of _______ ml eye drops, Sodium chloride required

$$= \frac{68}{10} \times \text{———} = \text{———} \text{ mg}$$

Label of Preparation:

PILOCARPINE NITRATE EYE DROPS			
Each 10 ml contains			
Pilocarpine nitrate	: 100.0 mg		
Sodium chloride	: 68.0 mg		
Solution of eye drops	: 10.0 ml		
Patient Name:		**Age:**	
Sex:		**Weight:**	
Dose: As directed by the physician.			
Mfg. Date:		**Exp. Date:**	
Batch No.:		**Price:**	
Prepared by:			

Date :___________   Marks : _________/10

EXPERIMENT NO. 90

- **Aim:** To prepare _______ ml pilocarpine eye drops.
- **Theory:** Eye drops must be freshly prepared aseptically and dispensed in previously sterilized container. A suitable fungistatic should be used in preparations liable to support the growth of moulds. For oily eye drops, the oily vehicle which has been previously sterilized by heating at 160°C for one hour must be used. Eye drops should be made approximately isotonic with lachrymal secretions by the addition of sodium chloride or other suitable substance. Care should be taken to avoid contamination during use.

  Uses: Glaucoma.

  Dose: As directed by physician.
- **Procedure:** Dissolve sodium chloride in solution of eye drops and prepare a solution. Add pilocarpine nitrate and dissolve it by shaking. Sterile by autoclave.
- **Storage:** Preserve in a well-closed container.

VIVA VOCE QUESTIONS

Q.1   What is eye glaucoma?

____

Q.2   How to manage glaucoma?

____

❖ ❖ ❖

Formulation Table:

Ingredients	Quantity required for 100 ml	Quantity required for _____ ml
Dextrose	5.0 g	_______ g
Water for injection	100.0 ml	_____ ml

Calculations:

Dextrose required to prepare 100 ml of injection =   5.0 g

So, for preparation of _______ ml injection, Dextrose required = $\dfrac{5}{100} \times$ ——— = ——— g

Label of Preparation:

DEXTROSE INJECTION			
Each 100 ml contains			
Dextrose : 5.0 g			
Water for injection : 100.0 ml			
Patient Name:		**Age:**	
Sex:		**Weight:**	
Dose: As directed by the physician.			
Mfg. Date:		**Exp. Date:**	
Batch No.:		**Price:**	
Prepared by:			

❖ ❖ ❖

Date :___________   Marks : _________/10

EXPERIMENT NO. 91

- **Aim:** To prepare _______ ml dextrose injection.

- **Theory:** Dextrose solution is a sterile solution of anhydrous dextrose or an equivalent quantity of dextrose monohydrated for parenteral solution. If the concentration of the solution is not reported, a 5% w/v solution should be prepared because it is isotonic with blood serum. The dextrose decomposes on heating. The rate of decomposition depends on sterilization temperature, duration of sterilization and presence of other substances. Decomposition of dextrose is reduced by adjusting the pH of injection between 3.5 to 6.5 using hydrochloric acid and also by avoiding overheating of injection. It should be cooled as quickly as possible after sterilization of the solution. Solution should not adhere to the neck of ampoules because it is converted in black form during the process of sealing. Injection should not be used if it contains a precipitate or any suspended particle.

  Uses: Source of energy.

  Dose: As directed by physician.

- **Procedure:** Dissolve the weighed quantity of dextrose in water for injection. Add sufficient water for injection to produce 100 ml. If necessary, filter the solution. 10 ml of solution is filled in each ampoule. The ampoules are sealed and sterilized immediately by autoclave.

- **Storage:** Preserve in a hermetically sealed ampoules.

VIVA VOCE QUESTIONS

Q.1   What is the use of dextrose injection?

____

Q.2   How to sterilize injection?

____

❖ ❖ ❖

Formulation Table:

Ingredients	Quantity required for 100 ml	Quantity required for _____ ml
Sodium chloride	0.9 g	_____ g
Water for injection	100.0 ml	_____ ml

Calculations:

Sodium chloride required to prepare 100 ml of injection = 0.9 g

So, for preparation of _______ ml injection, Sodium chloride required

$$= \frac{0.9}{100} \times \text{\_\_\_\_} = \text{\_\_\_\_} \; g$$

Label of Preparation:

SODIUM CHLORIDE INJECTION			
Each 100 ml contains			
Sodium chloride : 0.9 g			
Water for injection : 100.0 ml			
Patient Name:		**Age:**	
Sex:		**Weight:**	
Dose: As directed by the physician.			
Mfg. Date:		**Exp. Date:**	
Batch No.:		**Price:**	
Prepared by:			

❖❖❖

Date :___________   Marks : ________/10

EXPERIMENT NO. 92

- **Aim:** To prepare _______ ml sodium chloride injection.
- **Theory:** Injections are sterile products intended for administration of drugs by syringe and needle under the skin. The parenteral routes of the drug administration are indicated for less amount of drug required to reach at site of action.

  Uses: Electrolyte.

  Dose: As directed by physician.
- **Procedure:** Dissolve sodium chloride in sufficient quantity of water for injection. Add sufficient water for injection to produce 100 ml. If necessary, filter the solution. Fill the solution into the ampoules and seal them. Sterilize by autoclave as early as possible. Sterilization can also be done by filtration.
- **Storage:** Preserve in a hermetically sealed ampoules.

VIVA VOCE QUESTIONS

Q.1   What is the use of sodium chloride injection?

____

Q.2   How to sterilize injection?

____

❖ ❖ ❖

- **Formulation Table:**

Ingredients	Quantity required for 100 ml	Quantity required for _____ ml
Calcium gluconate	5.0 g	_____ g
Calcium D-saccharate	1.75 g	_____ g
Water for injection	100.0 ml	_____ ml

Calculations:

Calcium gluconate required to prepare 100 ml of injection = 5.0 g

So, for preparation of _______ ml injection, Calcium gluconate required

$$= \frac{5}{100} \times \text{------} = \text{------} \ g$$

Calcium D-saccharate required to prepare 100 ml of injection = 1.75 g

So, for preparation of _______ ml injection, Calcium D-saccharate required

$$= \frac{1.75}{100} \times \text{------} = \text{------} \ g$$

Label of Preparation:

<table>
<tr><td colspan="4" align="center">CALCIUM GLUCONATE INJECTION</td></tr>
<tr><td colspan="4">Each 100 ml contains</td></tr>
<tr><td colspan="4">Calcium gluconate   : 5.0 g</td></tr>
<tr><td colspan="4">Calcium D-saccharate : 1.75 g</td></tr>
<tr><td colspan="4">Water for injection   : 100.0 ml</td></tr>
<tr><td>Patient Name:</td><td></td><td>Age:</td><td></td></tr>
<tr><td>Sex:</td><td></td><td>Weight:</td><td></td></tr>
<tr><td colspan="4">Dose: As directed by the physician.</td></tr>
<tr><td>Mfg. Date:</td><td></td><td>Exp. Date:</td><td></td></tr>
<tr><td>Batch No.:</td><td></td><td>Price:</td><td></td></tr>
<tr><td colspan="4">Prepared by:</td></tr>
</table>

Date :___________   Marks : _________/10

EXPERIMENT NO. 93

- **Aim:** To prepare _______ ml calcium gluconate injection.
- **Theory:** Injections are sterile products intended for administration of drugs by syringe and needle under the skin. The parentral routes of the drug administration are indicated for less amount of drug required to reach at site of action.

  Uses: Fluid and Electrolyte.

  Dose: As directed by physician.
- **Procedure:** Dissolve calcium gluconate in water for injection. Add and dissolve calcium D-saccharate in solution. Adjust the pH 6.0 to 8.2 using 10% solution of sodium hydroxide. Filter through 0.45 µm membrane filter. Fill in 10 ml ampoules and seal them. Sterilize by autoclave at 121°C for 30 minutes.
- **Storage:** Preserve in a hermetically sealed ampoules.

VIVA VOCE QUESTIONS

Q.1   What is the use of calcium gluconate injection?

____

Q.2   How to sterilize injection?

____

❖ ❖ ❖

Formulation Table:

Ingredients	Quantity required for 100 ml	Quantity required for _____ ml
Potassium permanganate	0.1 g	_____ g
Purified water	100.0 ml	_____ ml

Calculations:

Potassium permanganate required to prepare 100 ml of douche = 0.1 g

So, for preparation of ____ ml douche, Potassium permanganate required

$$= \frac{0.1}{100} \times \underline{\quad} = \underline{\quad} \text{ ml}$$

Label of Preparation:

POTASSIUM PERMANGANATE DOUCHE			
Each 100 ml contains			
Potassium permanganate : 0.1 g			
Purified water : 100.0 ml			
Patient Name:		**Age:**	
Sex:		**Weight:**	
Dose: As directed by the physician.			
Mfg. Date:		**Exp. Date:**	
Batch No.:		**Price:**	
Prepared by:			

Date :__________   Marks : ________/10

EXPERIMENT NO. 94

- **Aim:** To prepare ________ ml potassium permanganate douche.
- **Theory:** A douche is an aqueous solution directed against a part or into a cavity of the body. Douches are most frequently dispensed in the form of a powder with directions for dissolving in a specified quantity of warm water. If powder or tablets are employed for this purpose, they must be completely soluble for this purpose, they must produce clear solution on dissolving.

  Uses: Antiseptic.

  Dose: As directed by physician.

- **Procedure:** Grind weighed amount of potassium permanganate with purified water using pestle mortar. Add more water and regrind. Allow undissolved crystals to settle and pour the supernatant into a conical flask. Filter through a clean sintered glass filter and make up the volume through filter.

- **Storage:** Preserve in a suitable container.

VIVA VOCE QUESTIONS

Q.1   What are douches?

____

Q.2   How to apply douches?

____

Q.3   How will you prepare douches?

____

❖ ❖ ❖

Formulation Table:

Ingredients	Quantity required for 100 ml	Quantity required for _____ ml
Alum	0.4 g	_____ g
Zinc sulphate	0.5 g	_____ g
Liquefied phenol	0.6 ml	_____ ml
Glycerin	12.5 ml	_____ ml
Purified water	100.0 ml	_____ ml

Calculations:

Alum required to prepare 100 ml of douche = 0.4 g

So, for preparation of _____ ml douche, Alum required = $\dfrac{0.4}{100} \times \underline{\quad} = \underline{\quad}$ g

Zinc sulphate required to prepare 100 ml of douche = 0.5 g

So, for preparation of _____ ml douche, Zinc sulphate required = $\dfrac{0.5}{100} \times \underline{\quad} = \underline{\quad}$ g

Liquefied phenol required to prepare 100 ml of douche = 0.6 ml

So, for preparation of _____ ml douche, Liquefied phenol required = $\dfrac{0.6}{100} \times \underline{\quad} = \underline{\quad}$ ml

Glycerin required to prepare 100 ml of douche = 12.5 ml

So, for preparation of _____ ml douche, Glycerin required = $\dfrac{12.5}{100} \times \underline{\quad} = \underline{\quad}$ ml

Label of Preparation:

ASTRINGENT DOUCHE		
Each 100 ml contains		
Alum : 0.4 g		
Zinc sulphate : 0.5 g		
Liquefied phenol : 0.6 ml		
Glycerin : 12.5 ml		
Purified water : 100.0 ml		
Patient Name:		**Age:**
Sex:		**Weight:**
Dose: As directed by the physician.		
Mfg. Date:		**Exp. Date:**
Batch No.:		**Price:**
Prepared by:		

Date :___________   Marks : ________/10

EXPERIMENT NO. 95

- **Aim:** To prepare _______ ml astringent douche.

- **Theory:** A douche is an aqueous solution directed against a part or into a cavity of the body. Douches are most frequently dispensed in the form of a powder with directions for dissolving in a specified quantity of warm water. If powder or tablets are employed for this purpose, they must be completely soluble for this purpose, they must produce clear solution on dissolving.

   Uses: Astringent.

   Dose: As directed by physician.

- **Procedure:** Grind weighed amount of alum with purified water using pestle mortar. Add zinc sulphate and dissolve. Gradually add liquefied phenol and glycerin and shake. Add sufficient purified water to produce 100 ml. If necessary, filter douche.

- **Storage:** Preserve in a suitable container.

VIVA VOCE QUESTIONS

Q.1   What are douches?

____

Q.2   How to apply douches?

____

Q.3   How will you prepare douches?

____

❖ ❖ ❖

Formulation Table:

Ingredients	Quantity required for 100 g	Quantity required for _____ g
Borax	12.0 g	_____ g
Glycerin	88.0 g	_____ g

Calculations:

Borax required to prepare 100 g of glycerite = 12.0 g

So, for preparation of _____ g glycerite, Borax required = $\dfrac{12}{100}$ × —— = —— g

Glycerin required to prepare 100 g of glycerite = 88.0 g

So, for preparation of _____ g glycerite, Glycerin required = $\dfrac{88}{100}$ × —— = —— g

Label of Preparation:

BORAX GLYCERITES			
Each 100 ml contains			
Borax : 12.0 g			
Glycerin : 88.0 g			
Patient Name:		**Age:**	
Sex:		**Weight:**	
Dose: As directed by the physician.			
Mfg. Date:		**Exp. Date:**	
Batch No.:		**Price:**	
Prepared by:			

Date :___________   Marks : _________/10

EXPERIMENT NO. 96

- **Aim:** To prepare _________ g borax gylcerin.

- **Theory:** Glycerites are solutions or mixtures of medicinal substances in glycerin. These formulations contain less than 50% of glycerin. Glycerin is important pharmaceutical solvent forming permanent and concentrated solutions. Glycerites are sweet in taste and do not become rancid during storage. Certain aqueous or non-aqueous preparations are used to remove wax from the ear. Glycerin is hygroscopic in nature and should be stored in air-tight closed container.

  Uses: Bacterostatic.

  Dose: As directed by physician.

- **Procedure:** Powder borax and pass it through sieve no. 80. Triturate fine powder of borax with glycerin. Warm the solution with constant stirring until borax is dissolved. Filter, if necessary.

- **Storage:** Preserve in a suitable container.

VIVA VOCE QUESTIONS

Q.1   What are glycerites?

____

Q.2   Why is borax used in the preprations?

____

Q.3   How it is used?

____

❖ ❖ ❖

Formulation Table:

Ingredients	Quantity required for 100 g	Quantity required for ______ g
Boric acid	31.0 g	______ g
Glycerin	69.0 g	______ g

Calculations:

Boric acid required to prepare 100 g of glycerite = 31.0 g

So, for preparation of ______ g glycerite, Boric acid required = $\dfrac{31}{100} \times$ —— = —— g

Glycerin required to prepare 100 g of glycerite = 69.0 g

So, for preparation of ______ g glycerite, Glycerin required = $\dfrac{69}{100} \times$ —— = —— g

Label of Preparation:

BORAX GLYCERITES			
Each 100 ml contains			
Boric acid　　: 31.0 g			
Glycerin　　 : 69.0 g			
Patient Name:		**Age:**	
Sex:		**Weight:**	
Dose: As directed by the physician.			
Mfg. Date:		**Exp. Date:**	
Batch No.:		**Price:**	
Prepared by:			

Date :___________   Marks : ________/10

EXPERIMENT NO. 97

- **Aim:** To prepare ________ g boric acid glycerin.

- **Theory:** Glycerites are solutions or mixtures of medicinal substances in glycerin. These formulations contain less than 50% of glycerin. Glycerin is important pharmaceutical solvent forming permanent and concentrated solutions. Glycerites are sweet in taste and do not become rancid during storage. Certain aqueous or non-aqueous preparations are used to remove wax from the ear. Glycerin is hygroscopic in nature and should be stored in air-tight closed container.

  Boric acid reacts with glycerin and forms boroglycerin. The rate of formation of boroglycerin is directly proportional to heat, but it should not be heated above 150°C. If heated above this temperature, the glycerin gets converted into acrolein, which is toxic in nature and colour of the preparation is changed to brownish.

  Uses: Antiseptic.

  Dose: As directed by physician.

- **Procedure:** Heat about half quantity of glycerin to a temperature of 140°C to 150°C in sand bath. Add boric acid and heat continuously with stirring until it dissolves. Evaporate at a temperature not exceeding 150°C until 20% of weight of the solution is reduced with continuous stirring. Add sufficient warm glycerin to produce the required weight.

VIVA VOCE QUESTIONS

Q.1   What are glycerites?

____

Q.2   Give pharmaceutical applications of boric acid?

____

Q.3   What is acrolein?

____

❖❖❖

Formulation Table:

Ingredients	Quantity required for 100 g	Quantity required for _____ g
Aluminium powder	20.0 g	_____ g
Zinc oxide	40.0 g	_____ g
Liquid paraffin	40.0 g	_____ g

Calculations:

Aluminium powder required to prepare 100 g of paste = 20.0 g

So, for preparation of _____ g paste, Aluminium powder required = $\dfrac{20}{100} \times$ —— = —— g

Zinc oxide required to prepare 100 g of paste = 40.0 g

So, for preparation of _____ g paste, Zinc oxide required = $\dfrac{40}{100} \times$ —— = —— g

Liquid paraffin required to prepare 100 g of paste = 40.0 g

So, for preparation of _____ g paste, Liquid paraffin required = $\dfrac{40}{100} \times$ —— = —— g

Label of Preparation:

<table>
<tr><td colspan="4" align="center">COMPOUND ALUMINIUM PASTE</td></tr>
<tr><td colspan="4">Each 100 g contains</td></tr>
<tr><td colspan="4">Aluminium powder : 20.0 g</td></tr>
<tr><td colspan="4">Zinc oxide : 40.0 g</td></tr>
<tr><td colspan="4">Liquid paraffin : 40.0 g</td></tr>
<tr><td>Patient Name:</td><td></td><td>Age:</td><td></td></tr>
<tr><td>Sex:</td><td></td><td>Weight:</td><td></td></tr>
<tr><td colspan="4">Dose: As directed by the physician.</td></tr>
<tr><td>Mfg. Date:</td><td></td><td>Exp. Date:</td><td></td></tr>
<tr><td>Batch No.:</td><td></td><td>Price:</td><td></td></tr>
<tr><td colspan="4">Prepared by:</td></tr>
</table>

Date :___________   Marks : _________/10

EXPERIMENT NO. 98

- **Aim:** To prepare _________ g compound aluminium paste.
- **Theory:** Pastes are semi-solid preparations, usually containing one or more medicaments in suitable base. They usually contain a high proportion of solids as compared to ointments. They are usually employed to apply medicaments to small localized area. Pastes should be supplied in collapsible tubes of metal or plastic which prevent the evaporation of the volatile additives.

  Uses: Mild astringent, protective and antiseptic.
- **Procedure:** Mix the aluminium powder and zinc oxide with liquid paraffin until smooth.
- **Storage:** Preserve in well-closed container.

VIVA VOCE QUESTIONS

Q.1   What are pastes?

____

Q.2   Why pastes are prepared?

____

❖ ❖ ❖

Formulation Table:

Ingredients	Quantity required for 100 g	Quantity required for _____ g
Zinc oxide	25.0 g	_____ g
Starch	25.0 g	_____ g
White soft paraffin	50.0 g	_____ g

Calculations:

Zinc oxide required to prepare 100 g of paste = 25.0 g

So, for preparation of _____ g paste, Zinc oxide required = $\dfrac{25}{100} \times$ ——— = ——— g

Starch required to prepare 100 g of paste = 25.0 g

So, for preparation of _____ g paste, Starch required = $\dfrac{25}{100} \times$ ——— = ——— g

White soft paraffin required to prepare 100 g of paste = 50.0 g

So, for preparation of _____ g paste, White soft paraffin required = $\dfrac{50}{100} \times$ ——— = ——— g

Label of Preparation:

COMPOUND ZINCPASTE			
Each 100 g contains			
Zinc oxide : 25.0 g			
Starch : 25.0 g			
White soft paraffin : 50.0 g			
Patient Name:		**Age:**	
Sex:		**Weight:**	
Dose: As directed by the physician.			
Mfg. Date:		**Exp. Date:**	
Batch No.:		**Price:**	
Prepared by:			

Date :___________   Marks : ________/10

EXPERIMENT NO. 99

- **Aim:** To prepare _________ g compound zinc paste.
- **Theory:** Pastes are semi-solid preparations, usually containing one or more medicaments in suitable base. They usually contain a high proportion of solids as compared to ointments. They are usually employed to apply medicaments to small localized area. Pastes should be supplied in collapsible tubes of metal or plastic which prevent the evaporation of the volatile additives.

  Uses: Astringent, protective and antiseptic.
- **Procedure:** Melt white soft paraffin in a glass container. Incorporate zinc oxide and starch and stir until cold.
- **Storage:** Preserve in well-closed container.

VIVA VOCE QUESTIONS

Q.1   What is the difference between pastes and ointments?

____

Q.2   What are the applications of paste?

____

❖ ❖ ❖

Formulation Table:

Ingredients	Quantity required for 100 g	Quantity required for _____ g
Strong coal tar solution	7.5 ml	_____ ml
Compound zinc paste	100.0 g	_____ g

Calculations:

Strong coal tar solution required to prepare 100 g of paste = 7.5 ml

So, for preparation of _____ g paste, Strong coal tar solution required

$$= \frac{75}{100} \times \text{------} = \text{------ ml}$$

Compound zinc paste required to prepare 100 g of paste = 100.0 g

So, for preparation of _____ g paste, Compound zinc paste required

$$= \frac{100}{100} \times \text{------} = \text{------ g}$$

Label of Preparation:

COAL TAR PASTE			
Each 100 g contains			
Strong coal tar solution : 7.5 ml			
Compound zinc paste : 100.0 g			
Patient Name:		**Age:**	
Sex:		**Weight:**	
Dose: As directed by the physician.			
Mfg. Date:		**Exp. Date:**	
Batch No.:		**Price:**	
Prepared by:			

Date :___________   Marks : _________/10

EXPERIMENT NO. 100

- **AIM:** To prepare _________ g coal tar paste.

- **Theory:** Pastes are semi-solid preparations, usually containing one or more medicaments in suitable base. They usually contain a high proportion of solids as compared to ointments. They are usually employed to apply medicaments to small localized area. Pastes should be supplied in collapsible tubes of metal or plastic which prevent the evaporation of the volatile additives.

  Uses: Protective.

- **Procedure:** Prepare strong coal tar solution and compound zinc paste. Triturate strong coal tar solution with a portion of the compound zinc paste until smooth. Gradually add the remaining amount of the compound zinc paste.

- **Storage:** Preserve in well-closed container.

VIVA VOCE QUESTIONS

Q.1   What is the difference between pastes and gels?

____

Q.2   What are the applications of pastes?

____

❖ ❖ ❖

NOTES

NOTES

NOTES

NOTES